Crowdsourced Health

Crowdsourced Health

How What You Do on the Internet Will Improve Medicine

Elad Yom-Tov

The MIT Press
Cambridge, Massachusetts
London, England

Set in Stone Sans and Stone Serif by Toppan Best-set Premedia Limited. Printed and bound in the United States of America.

Library of Congress Cataloging-in-Publication Data

Names: Yom-Tov, Elad, author.
Title: Crowdsourced health : how what you do on the Internet will improve medicine / Elad Yom-Tov.
Description: Cambridge, MA : The MIT Press, [2015] | Includes bibliographical references and index.
Identifiers: LCCN 2015038415 | ISBN 9780262034500 (hardcover : alk. paper)
Subjects: | MESH: Crowdsourcing. | Data Mining. | Biomedical Research. | Internet.
Classification: LCC R858 | NLM W 26.55.I4 | DDC 610.285–dc23 LC record available at http://lccn.loc.gov/2015038415

10 9 8 7 6 5 4 3 2 1

To my parents, Shlomith (RIP) and Yoram, who taught me to inquire. To Galit and the boys.

Contents

Acknowledgments

I have had opportunities to work with many talented scientists in the course of my work. Some are mentioned in this book, and I am indebted to them all for what they taught me during our work together, and for the privilege of working with them.

I was, and still am, fortunate to have worked at companies that value long-term research. My managers at these companies, Evgeniy Gabrilovich, Andrei Broder, and Jennifer Chayes, challenged me with their questions and ideas to look farther and deeper. One could not ask for better research managers and colleagues.

Finally, I am thankful to the editors at the MIT Press and to Jennifer Collins, who improved the manuscript greatly.

Introduction

Beginnings

One gray autumn New York morning I received an email message from my mother. It was with a bunch of other messages that had arrived during the night, and it had no subject line. With my mother, a lack of a subject line was always a bad sign, because it meant that she could not put the subject into words. I left that message for last, and when I finally read it my fears were confirmed. A routine blood test had resulted in a diagnosis of cancer. It was not an especially bad cancer, she wrote, but the alternatives for treatment ranged from the benign wait-and-see option to the awful. That day, at the office, I paced to and fro. I was 5,000 miles away from my parents, and I felt pretty useless. However, I am a computer scientist, so I figured I should go online and find what was known about her condition. Later that moment of unknowing would come back to me as the beginning of the research that would lead to this book.

Even though I consider myself quite savvy in using search engines, and even building them is one part of my job, that day was a frustrating experience. Many websites discussed such things as diagnosis of a disease and what one can expect from your doctor. This information was irrelevant, since it was geared to patients or to people whose diagnosis was yet unknown. Worse, most Web pages that discussed the possible outcomes of the disease gave all the options for outcomes as if they were equally likely, though even for me, a layperson, that seemed improbable.

A few days later, when I got used to the idea, and when more tests had revealed that the situation was not as bad as my family and I initially feared, I began thinking about my experience and how it could be improved. This was not altogether a new field for me. At the time I was working for the research arm of the Internet giant Yahoo, where I specialized in improving Yahoo's search engine. But going beyond improving a search engine, for several months I had been thinking about a more general question: Since so many people use the Internet nowadays, and since Internet companies collect data that are generated while people use the Internet, could we learn something new and interesting about medicine—something that would be hard to learn in other ways? Could medical doctors learn something useful from how I and many thousands of other people learn about cancer? Could it improve how doctors communicate with patients? Could it provide new insights that might change how patients are treated?

How can Internet data assist your physician?

Internet data mirror our offline behavior, in the sense that many of our actions in the physical world are manifested by some online data. Consider your last vacation. Before you decided where to go, you may have searched for hotels, and later uploaded photos of that vacation to your favorite social network, or tweeted about a restaurant that served an unforgettable dish. These actions all create online data that tell a story about your offline behavior. But Internet data have additional advantages. First, they are generated almost continuously, whereas medical data usually are created only when you visit a doctor or undergo a medical test. Second, in some cases (which will be discussed in chapter 2) people feel more at ease in sharing their most sensitive questions online than with their doctor. Finally, Internet data offer a window into online activities that may be of medical importance, as I will discuss in chapter 4.

The main claim of this book is that, because Internet data closely follows our behavior offline, Internet data can change how medical research is done, and have already begun doing so. Gaining insights from Internet data requires collaboration between medical researchers and computer scientists, and the results of such collaborations can provide insights not otherwise available. Research using these data will not replace clinical trials or other means of conducting medical research. Instead, this research can augment traditional tools to shed light on questions that were difficult to answer previously. Internet data allow, to some extent, the creation of a new kind of science.

One of my main reasons for writing this book is that I hope it will spawn new ideas for medical research. Thus far we have only scratched the surface of what is possible; however, a lot of data are being collected, and those data can and should be put to good use.

This book is the culmination of several years of work in this new area of investigation by myself and others. Work that began, for me, with that introspective observation on how people learn about a disease. These efforts show that the behavior of people is a tremendously useful source of data for learning about human health and medicine. It certainly does not replace more traditional ways of medical research, but it augments such research in areas where information is hard to glean.

In the past several years researchers have found new side effects of medical drugs, examined the association between being overweight or underweight and being bullied, studied the information needs of cancer patients and their families, sought insights into the world of anorexia sufferers, and even found a link between perceptions of anorexia and how underweight celebrities are portrayed in the media. Questions about all these matters would have been difficult or impossible to answer with conventional tools of medical research. These investigations have convinced me that there are four main areas where the use of Internet data has advantages over traditional medical tools and data. Such advantages are gained where it is hard or impossible to collect unbiased data in the physical world, when more sensitive measurements are needed than those that are traditionally afforded by medical information, when people have difficulty reporting the data researchers need to validate their hypotheses, or when most of the activity happens online. Therefore, after describing why Internet data are so abundant and how they are collected, I will discuss some of the knowledge to be gained in each of these areas.

Throughout the book, I describe how those of us who are conducting research in the area, that recently has come to be referred to as "data science", approach problems and solve them. We have a variety of tools at our disposal, including advanced statistics, studies of users, online questionnaires, and billions of search-engine queries and social-media postings. Because most of these tools are unknown to the wider public, I show how they can be utilized to gain insights into human behavior.

This book is written for medical researchers and practitioners, who, I believe, should be made aware of the advantages afforded by Internet data and of the likelihood that such data can help them improve health by shining light on areas that otherwise are difficult to investigate. This book is also intended for all who are interested in interdisciplinary research that links seemingly disparate fields of knowledge. It is my hope that the research described here will trigger new ideas about how to better provide medicine using the insights garnered from Internet data. Arthur C. Clarke's third "law" states that any sufficiently advanced technology is indistinguishable from magic. I hope that at least some of the findings presented in this book will initially appear to be magic even to readers who specialize in medicine or computer science, but that understanding how they came about will help spawn new advances. We have only scratched the surface of what is possible with Internet data.

An idea is born

When I give talks about my work, mostly at universities and at academic conferences, I usually describe two or three of the projects I describe in this book. If the talk is successful, someone will raise their hand during the talk, or come to the podium after it, and say something like "Have you considered looking at this other problem?" Sometimes it is a medical problem that this person has encountered, and sometimes it is one that he has a personal interest in. In many cases, the person who raised the subject is somewhat of an expert on it. Such was the case with my work on anorexia, which began with a comment made by a graduate student after a talk I gave at the Georgia Institute of Technology. A few years later, the idea to look at behaviors that are precursor to disease started with discussions over coffee after a lecture at University College London.

Often research is spawned by seemingly random ideas. At other times it begins with a computer scientist noticing interesting quirks in some data or feeling that an interesting implication might be drawn from these data. In chapter 2 we will see such a case, which began when Dan Pelleg, then my colleague at Yahoo Research, found about 80,000 questions on Yahoo Answers such as "Am I fat?" (or thin, or underweight, or obese) and giving the asker's age, gender, weight, and height.

Once an idea is born, developing it is an interesting process in and of itself. It begins by bridging the language gap between computer scientists and medical experts. Words can mean very different things in different professions, and at first it is necessary to clarify what each side means. Then there is a dialogue about what is interesting and what is possible. My friend Yishai Ofran, a hematologist, once came to me with an epidemiological question that he thought would be easy for me to answer: Do some life-changing events, such as an ugly divorce or a painful layoff from a job, increase the likelihood of cancer? I tried to answer that question using the data I had, but still have not been able to do so.

In my attempt to answer Yishai's question, I began looking at whether I could identify people who had recently been diagnosed with cancer according to the questions they submitted to the Yahoo search engine. Being able to do identify these people was not very useful for Yishai, but then I showed him what people wanted to know in the first few days after they were diagnosed, and that got both of us interested in the information needs of patients and their friends soon after patients are told that they have cancer. You can read about that work, and how we were able to validate a 40-year-old psychological model, in chapter 5.

The best data collection, the worst data collection

To paraphrase Dickens,[1] large-scale data collection by Internet providers and website operators is both a sign of the age of foolishness and a sign of the age of wisdom. Internet providers and website operators can be a threat to our privacy, but they can also provide insights into people's behavior that never were available before. Properly used, these data are a real boon to medical research.

Large-scale data collection has, in recent times, earned a bad name for itself. Depending on where in the world you live and whether you are more worried about industry's collecting data or about government's hoarding data, you may have heard about the U.S. National Security Agency's collection of data from many of the worlds' Internet companies,[2] about how Facebook knows about the lives of about one sixth of the worlds' population, or how Google was fined for illegally collecting data.[3] Such excesses aside, most Internet companies collect vast amounts of data so as to provide their services and to improve them. A search-engine operator such as Google or Bing needs, at a minimum, to store an up-to-date copy of the entire (visible) Internet, including every page it might show as a result to any query from a person anywhere. In order to serve the right pages, a search-engine operator usually also stores data on how users interacted with the search engine—what pages they clicked on (and therefore, perhaps, thought useful) and which pages they did not click on. These are vast amounts of data, and the fact that they are growing at an astounding rate should be of concern to anyone who worries about personal privacy.

The other side of the coin is that large-scale data collection provides an opportunity to improve peoples' health in a direct and quantitatively measureable manner. In essence, data you generate online help to improve the health of many other people while helping improve yours. For example (as we will see in chapter 4), when people search for information on adverse reactions they are experiencing from the drugs they take, their searches can assist in identifying previously unknown adverse reactions.

The term *crowdsourcing* was coined in 2005 by Jeff Howe and Mark Robinson, two editors at *Wired*. They combined the words "crowd" and "outsourcing" to describe how companies began taking tasks previously performed by their employees and giving these tasks to other people, usually through some mechanism of open calls. The *Oxford English Dictionary* defines crowdsourcing as "the practice of obtaining information or input into a task … by enlisting the services of a large number of people … typically via the Internet." Strictly speaking, Internet data (whether or not related to health) are not explicitly solicited from people who create them. Nevertheless, I consider the use of contributions made by a large number of people to solve problems related to health a new facet of crowdsourcing.

In the past a large portion of health-related data came from hospitals and clinics, but such data reflect only certain aspects of people's health—mostly those aspects that represent sickness. With Internet data we can observe the more mundane sides of life and the facets of health that do not require medical attention. Internet data can help to improve the well-being of entire populations. The health of a population can be enhanced through the contributions of data made by each person in it.

The story of how large-scale data collection can be highly beneficial to human health is worth telling. It is told in the pages of this book.

1 Our Data, Ourselves

In May 2012 I gave a talk at the renowned Xerox PARC Forum on some of the work described in this book, showing how a range of medical questions can be addressed through analysis of Internet data. After the talk, one of the people who came to ask questions identified himself as an engineer working for one of Silicon Valley's best-known companies. He asked me about our users' privacy, and I began to explain how we are careful to maintain that privacy, but he cut me short. "You don't understand," he said. "I see people in my company using this data all the time, but it's the first time I've seen it put to good use."

This book builds on the recent availability of massive amounts of data collected while people use the Internet for a variety of tasks, and its fruits are the unprecedented possibilities to gain medical insights from very large populations of people. My goal in this book is to show how these data can enable us to learn about our health and medicine without compromising our individual privacy.

Before delving into how we can learn about people's health from behavioral data on the Internet, this chapter describes how and why these data are generated. We will begin with how people use the Internet for anything ranging from work to pleasure, from search engines to social networking. While using the Internet, people generate a wealth of data. We will see some examples of these data and the opportunity they create for research. Equally important, we will look at some of the hazards to privacy that go hand in hand with the collection of behavioral data, and how these hazards can be mitigated by proper care in the handling of such data.

The gathering of data about people's behavior on the Web is a fairly recent phenomenon. Like other significant advances in technology, it has the promise to deliver both good and evil. Speaking in 1946, Bernard Baruch told the UN Atomic Energy Commission: "Science has taught us how to put the atom to work. But to make it work for good instead of for evil lies in the domain dealing with the principles of human duty. We are now facing a problem more of ethics than physics."[1] We are in a similar situation today with regard to data. Data can be used for ignoble causes that can infringe on our privacy and our freedom, but also, as I hope to convince you, can be used in ways that will improve individual and public health.

The data we generate during our online activities

In the United States, 85 percent of adults use the Internet, and most of them use it daily,[2] most commonly to search for information, send and receive email messages, check the weather, or just pass the time.[3] In the past, conducting research for a scientific paper or hanging out with friends were activities that left little permanent record of their happening, except perhaps the record of the books I borrowed from a library or in the memory of the friends I met. Comparable activities performed online leave long-lasting impressions, because they are recorded on the servers of Facebook, Google, and almost any other website operator I visit.

Throughout this book I will refer to data of the latter sort as "Internet data." Researchers often describe such data as "Internet behavioral data" or "user-generated content." These descriptions are meant to impart the understanding that the data were created by individuals (as opposed to, say, operators of news channels) and are primarily created and accessed online. This delineation was never clear cut, and is becoming fuzzier as more and more of our leisure and work time is spent on the Internet. Are data created through the use of apps on our cellular phones considered "Internet data"? I don't think so, but other researchers may beg to differ. Do the data transmitted to the Internet by my fitness tracker during my morning jog become "Internet data"? Again, I don't think so, but others may disagree. On the other hand, I tend to regard search-engine queries as user-generated data, whereas scientists who study social media probably would not. Therefore, in most portions of this book the reader should take the term "Internet data" in the broad sense.

The amounts of data that are generated and stored during our use of the Internet are staggering. In December 2012, in the United States alone, an estimated 17.6 billion queries were made to Internet search engines, mostly to Google, Bing, and Yahoo.[4] That amounts to about 50 queries per person (man, woman, or child). During that month, Facebook collected about 15 petabytes (15,000 terabytes, or 15 million gigabytes) of data,[5] which amounts to approximately 2,150 bytes—roughly equivalent to an old-fashioned letter—for every human in the world. It is estimated that Amazon used between 500,000 and 5.6 million computers to collect and process data on its public computing platform.[6]

The use of Internet search engines is one of the most common activities online. Although the average length of a query typed into a Web browser's search box has long been three words,[7] search-engine operators receive much more information with each query. First, each search engine knows what results were returned in response to the query. The "ten blue links" include the results documents that have been traditionally associated with search engines but more recently also include images, videos, news results, and information summaries that search engines now show. Usually, search engines also log which of the links were clicked and how long a user stayed on the page after clicking on it. The latter is an important signal of how relevant the information on the page is to the user.

An additional signal that many search engines record is the general location of the user. Especially in the United States, location gives powerful clues about the user's demographic characteristics, income, and even voting pattern.

What do I mean when I query "Second Avenue Deli"? Am I looking for the telephone number of a deli on 2nd Avenue, close to where I am now, or for the website of a New York establishment by that name? It is hard to guess the intention of a user from three words, and so the additional data associated with the query are collected for one primary reason: to improve the search engine so that it provides better answers to the user by predicting his or her intention and matching it to the most relevant documents. A secondary reason for collecting the data is to enable advertisers to tailor their advertisements to users, but that is beyond the scope of this book.

Knowing which documents were favored by different people, even in response to the same query, can help in tailoring the information that will be provided. This process, called *personalization*, can depend on various pieces of information. For example, we now know that the readability of a page (that is, how "highbrow" the language in it is) strongly influences which people will like the page. Thus, if a good result for some query is a Wikipedia page, it is better to provide certain people with the regular English-language edition of Wikipedia, whereas others would be better served by the corresponding simplified Wikipedia page, written using 1,000 common English words.

Once collected, data can be used in ways not always originally imagined. The retail-store chain Target, for example, lets people create baby registries so that family members and friends can buy gifts for new parents. These registries can then be linked to purchases made at Target stores by the parents before and throughout the pregnancy. As Charles Duhigg of the *New York Times* reported,[8] this is exactly what one of Target's statisticians did, finding, for example, that "women on the baby registry were buying larger quantities of unscented lotion around the beginning of their second trimester." This enabled Target to predict which of its female customers are pregnant simply by monitoring their purchases, and then to send them precisely timed marketing offers. As Target found, this can sometimes work too well: Duhigg tells the story of an angry father who walked into a Target store complaining that his high-school-age daughter had received advertisements for baby cloths and cribs, wondering "Are you trying to encourage her to get pregnant?" Though this could have been a classification error by an automatic system, in this case the father apologized a few weeks later: "I had a talk with my daughter. It turns out there's been some activities in my house I haven't been completely aware of. She's due in August." The shopping activities of the daughter had indeed pinpointed the fact that she was pregnant, even if at the time she may not have known it herself. Innocuous information on her shopping led Target to infer something that was never intended by her, and of a very sensitive nature at that.

Real-world information from digital data

On average, people make from five to eight searches a day.[9] That is not a huge number, but it still makes search-engine queries a rich source of information on people's activities both in the virtual world and in the physical world.

In the physical world, Lars Backstrom and his colleagues[10] at Yahoo Research and at Cornell University found that when they examined the places people were querying from they could easily show the path of hurricanes, the coverage of cell-phone companies, and the locations of the fan bases of baseball teams. Intuitively, the closer people were to the path of the hurricane, the more likely they were to query about it. By tracking the location of people who were querying for information about a specific hurricane, the path of the hurricane could be identified. Of course, there are better ways to find a hurricane's path, or to figure out the coverage of a cell-phone company, but these cases illustrate the possibility of obtaining information about the physical world from the virtual one.

A more practical demonstration of these capabilities was developed in earthquake-prone Japan. Using the micro-blog service Twitter, which also tracks the location of some users, Takeshi Sakaki and his colleagues[11] at the University of Tokyo were able to warn of earthquakes within one minute of their beginning, whereas the Japan Meteorological Agency typically takes six minutes to report a quake.

In the medical domain, tracking influenza epidemics using search-engine logs has been a topic of intensive research since about 2006. This is because tens of millions of people contract influenza each year, and an estimated 250,000–500,000 people die from it. Moreover, the symptoms associated with influenza are well known. Thus, the combination of a large patient group and clear set of symptoms made influenza a prime target for what has since been called "infodemiology."[12]

Initial efforts at tracking influenza using Internet data began not with search logs themselves but with advertisements placed by search engines next to the results of searches. According to Gunther Eysenbach, who conducted this research, "while Google normally does not provide detailed logs [for searches] conducted on its sites[,] it does provide rather detailed statistics for advertisers who "buy" (or rather bid for) certain keywords in … its advertising program." Gunther spent all of $365.64 to place ads on Google and track the number of people in Canada who queried for "flu" or "flu symptoms," and showed that it had an excellent correlation with epidemiological information collected by the official Public Health Agency of Canada (which relies on reports from a group of physicians, probably at a much higher cost than Gunther had to pay).[13]

Gunther was looking at the total prevalence of influenza in Canada. A later attempt at tracking this disease had a much more fine-grained approach, which also relied on actual query data, not ads. Jeremy Ginsberg and his colleagues at Google had access to Google's search logs (first in the United States, later globally), and to the location of users. In their *Nature* paper they show that the number of influenza-related searches correlated with information from visits to physicians, even at a regional level.[14]

Recently, however, the resulting product, Google Flu Trends, proved to be inaccurate because of higher-than-average media interest in the flu season. Google overestimated the prevalence of influenza[15] simply because people heard on the news that there is an influenza epidemic and then went online to search for information about it. Oversights in the design of a complicated system such as Google Flu Trends are inevitable, yet the system provides evidence of both the promise and the limitations of using online data to track diseases.

Internet data and threats to privacy

The fact that search-engine logs are revealing of people's interests is both their most useful and their most disturbing aspect. In fact, even data which has undergone a process of anonymization is no guarantee of complete anonymity. A case in point is the (intentional) leak of search data from AOL.

Every researcher who works with search-engine logs knows the following story: On August 4, 2006, Abdur Chowdhury, then AOL's chief scientist, released a log of 20 million searches from about 650,000 anonymized users. The anonymization was done by assigning a number to each user, under the assumption that, although all searches of the same user could be identified, users themselves would remain anonymous. The log was released for use in research, because AOL did not have sufficient resources to conduct its own research in house. Alas, within three days AOL recognized its mistake and removed the log. By then, so many copies had been made that it is still easy to obtain the data today.

The mistake was that, even though users were anonymized, search-engine logs are still very revealing. For example, user 4417749 searched for "landscapers in Lilburn, Ga," which hinted that she lived in Lilburn, Georgia (a town with a population of about 11,000), that she had a dog (as was evident from her query "dog that urinates on everything"), and that she probably was about 60 years old (she was looking for "60 single men"). It did not take long for the *New York Times'* reporter to identify her as Thelma Arnold, a 62-year-old widow from Lilburn.[16]

Many years later, data from the AOL query log are still being used. In 2012, for example, Google Scholar, a search engine for academic papers, listed 1,150 papers that mentioned the AOL query log. In her book *The Immortal life of Henrietta Lacks*, Rebecca Skloot documents how, more than 50 years after Lacks' death, cancerous cells from her tumors are still used for research in biology labs around the world. Similarly, Thelma Arnold's data are still being used for research, and she cannot get those data deleted. This is a stark lesson in the dangers of digital data: once stored, digital data cannot be "unstored."

AOL is by no means a unique example. In 2010 the organizers of a scientific conference released data from Flickr, a photo-sharing website. The data, consisting of links between anonymized Flickr users, were released so that people could compete on predicting (for a different subset of the data) which users would be "friends" on the website. Instead of tackling that problem as the organizers of the conference had planned, Arvind Narayanan and his students at Princeton University decided to undertake a slightly different task: they mapped the anonymized data back to the website and then found which users were linked on the actual website.[17]

Even people who are conscious of their privacy are at risk of losing it through the action of friends who are less conscious of privacy than they are. Carter Jernigan and Behram Mistree[18] noticed that, on average, only 0.7 percent of a heterosexual man's Facebook friends are gay men, but that typically 4.6 percent of the friends of a man who identifies as gay are gay men.

Using this simple observation, they were able to predict the sexual orientations of MIT students with a high accuracy, even when those students did not reveal their sexual preferences.

Thus, the data we leave on the Web when we "surf" are highly revealing of who we are and what we are. Anonymity of data is no guarantee of complete anonymity.

Can studies which use Internet data be done ethically?

Another critical question, intricately intertwined with privacy, concerns ethics: Should it be lawful to use Internet data in the pursuit of medical knowledge, even though a large portion of Internet data is generated for purposes other than medical research?

Over the years, too many scientific studies had treated humans so egregiously that it was obvious ethical standards of research should be implemented to reduce, if not eliminate, violations of basic human dignity in scientific research. Some of the worst examples of such research were horrific Nazi experiments on Jewish and other prisoners before and during World War II and similar experiments on Chinese citizens by the Japanese Army's Unit 731. In the United States, the Tuskegee syphilis experiment, conducted between 1932 and 1972, observed the progression of syphilis in African-American men without treating it, even though an effective treatment was available. Indeed, participants were not even told that they had the disease.

Such experiments led to the formation, in many countries,[19] of Institutional Review Boards (IRBs)—committees tasked with evaluating experiments that deal with human subjects, evaluating the experiments both before and during their execution. The goal of IRBs is to conduct a risk-benefit analysis and decide if the experiments can be performed without overly compromising human rights and welfare. IRBs want to protect humans from physical and psychological harm by ensuring that experimenters follow three primary principles: respect for the people participating in the experiment, beneficence i.e., that the experimenter acts in the best interest of the participant, and justice which in this case means fairness and equality among patients.[20]

By and large, IRBs are part and parcel of any university-run experiment that involves humans. Moreover, in the United States any experiment that forms the basis for an application to the Food and Drug Administration requires prior approval by an IRB. Therefore, any drug or medical device that is approved for use in the U.S. will have been tested in an IRB-approved experiment.

Internet companies, however, are not universities and usually are not applying for a license from the FDA. Therefore, a large part of Internet research is not subject to IRB oversight or approval. This was made very clear in late 2013 when a group of researchers published a paper in the *Proceedings of the National Academy of Sciences* titled "Experimental evidence of massive-scale emotional contagion through social networks," or, as *Slate* called it "Facebook's unethical experiment."[21] The paper detailed an experiment, carried out during one week in 2012, in which the Facebook "walls," or news feeds, of nearly 700,000 people were reordered by Facebook researchers so that some users saw at the top of their feeds slightly more upbeat posts by their friends while others saw slightly more pessimistic ones. The researchers wanted to see if such differences would cause a change in the mood of these people.[22] The experiment had some positive results and some negative ones. Yes, people who were exposed to downbeat sentiment were more likely to post more cheerless posts, and vice versa. However, whether that reflected their own moods or just their willingness to conform to their environment was not clear. On the flip side, the number of pessimistic posts made by each user who saw downbeat posts by his friends was small. The largest effect was two hundredths of a standard deviation. This is one of the reasons why such a large sample size was needed: Measuring tiny effects requires very large populations in order to yield a significant result.

Perhaps the more interesting part of the aforementioned experiment happened after the results of the experiment had been published. Several news outlets characterized the experiment as "making [Facebook] users sad," and thus possibly harming these users. They further claimed that such research required approval by an IRB, and that the fact that the research in question had not been approved by an IRB (though in a sense it had been) indicated a violation of ethical standards. I think this study exemplifies the difficulty that Internet data studies pose, especially with regard to health, and for that reason I would like to dwell on that study a little.

As I noted above, officially Facebook did not require IRB approval, because it isn't a university and wasn't seeking FDA approval. Two of the study's authors were, however, affiliated with Cornell University. The members of Cornell's IRB considered whether the study required their approval and decided that it did not, because the study was to be conducted at Facebook, not at Cornell. Such formalities may justly cause us to feel uneasy, so let's assume that Facebook would have sought IRB approval. Would Facebook have gotten it?

Interestingly, the answer is "probably yes," even though Facebook did not obtain explicit consent from the participants, as is done for the vast majority of medical research. First, when users join Facebook they agree to participate in research. The clause that allows the use of data from an Internet website to be used for research appears in many of the "Terms of Use" we agree to when we join a website. Second, though Facebook manipulated people's news feeds, it merely changed the order in which items were shown. A user who scrolled down far enough would have seen all the posts anyway. Changing the ordering of posts is something Facebook probably does every day so as to find more engaging ways of presenting information, thus getting people to use Facebook more. An IRB would probably consider this manipulation no different from all the other ways that order is changed, no better and no worse.

In the wider scheme of things, Internet companies continually experiment to improve their products.[23] This is one of the reasons these services are so addictive and so successful.[24] The only way search engines such as Google and Bing can improve is by tweaking their results and then seeing if most people like the changes. In fact, whenever you use a search engine, you are probably participating in any number of experiments testing the colors that are used to display the results,[25] the fonts, and the pages served. If we allow such experimentation (and we have to allow them in order for a search engine to operate), shouldn't we allow the use of data collected from such experiments to be used for medical research?

This is not a simple question to answer, since there are many shades to the collection of these data. We can use data collected for other reasons (for example, simply when users post information or issue queries to a search engine), and we can try to elicit data, as in the Facebook study or in other studies that tried to cause users to behave in a certain manner by showing (or refraining to show) information. We can try to steer people away from harmful behavior or toward more beneficial behavior. We can combine data from multiple sources or use data from a single source, the latter making it narrower and less intrusive. We can use identifiable data, or aggregated, anonymized data. All these cases are not equal, and outside of the IRB system we do not have a good process by which to decide which studies should be done and which should not.

To put this challenge in more concrete terms, most people would agree that if a pharmaceutical company shows advertisements online to try and persuade people to use their product, this would not require IRB approval, even if the advertisements were using scare tactics. Similarly, we do not bar anti-vaccination advocates from advertising their ideas, though we know that they have harmful effects.[26] Should we therefore require IRB approval for studies that use online advertisements to encourage anorexics to seek help? Should we require IRB approval for studies that try to elicit public sentiment toward vaccines, because they may cause people to change their opinion, simply because of the way a question is asked?

My personal view is that as a researcher I am better off consulting a larger group of people, be they ethicists or simply people with differing views, even if I am not officially obligated to do so. For the purpose of a consultation an IRB is a valuable group of people, and my current employer, Microsoft, maintains such an IRB. However, as an industry we are still grappling with the question of ethics in all the manifestations of the various experiments which use Internet data.

As was eloquently summarized by Michelle Meyer in *Wired*,[27] "it turns out that those [human subject research] laws don't apply to the [Facebook] study, and even if they did, it could have been approved, perhaps with some tweaks. … We can certainly have a conversation about the appropriateness of Facebook-like manipulations, data mining, and other 21st-century practices. But so long as we allow private entities to engage freely in these practices, we ought not to unduly restrain academics trying to determine their effects. ... IRBs make it impossible to study the effects of appeals that carry the same intensity of fear as real-world appeals to which people are exposed routinely, and on a mass scale, with unknown consequences. That doesn't make a lot of sense. What corporations can do at will to serve their bottom line, and non-profits can do to serve their cause, we shouldn't make (even) harder—or impossible—for those seeking to produce generalizable knowledge to do."[28]

In the following chapters we will analyze these sensitive data, knowing full well that they are sensitive and taking care to keep the people we observe anonymous. The data are always anonymized before we even received them, but since that is not enough to maintain the complete privacy of our users we always try to examine the data in aggregate. Therefore, we will rarely look at what user 4417749 is searching for, preferring to ask "How many users asked about the drug Lipitor, and then asked about chest pain?"

In addition, privacy is easier to compromise when we link data from different sources. For example, we might not know the identity of a specific user of a search engine user, but if we somehow matched his searches to a Facebook profile we would immediately know his name and possibly his address. Therefore, we try not to make such links (or "joins," as they are called in the industry).

Nevertheless, I believe that Internet data should be used, with appropriate privacy safeguards, because of the unprecedented insights they can provide into peoples' behaviors and experiences. As Iain Buchan noted in a panel discussion at the 2013 Microsoft Machine Learning Summit, we need to "discuss privacy thoroughly, but always in a risk-benefit context, never in a risk-only context, because that is completely artificial." In our case, context is the betterment of human health, surely a noble cause.

How Internet data can be of use in medical research

Our work has suggested that there are several areas in which Internet data are useful and, at times, superior to data collected by traditional means.

First, our ability to identify searches as coming from the same person enables us to make associations that are hard for people to make. As we will see in chapter 4, people are very good at identifying adverse reactions to medicines they began to take a few days ago, but are very bad at linking medicines to adverse reactions that take a longer time to appear. Using search-engine logs lets us do the linking, and this ability brings big benefits for consumer safety.

Second, sometimes passive, non-intrusive observation such as observation derived from Internet data is the only practicable way to collect data. Researchers who tried to track what parents of children who have cancer go through in the first few weeks after diagnosis found that many would not participate in the study, or would not complete it, mostly because they were (not surprisingly) "feeling overwhelmed" by the news and what they had to do about it. Using search data to conduct similar studies can be achieved by observing peoples' searches, though because we do not have a way to be sure that we are observing patients, caregivers, or friends we had to develop methods to make sure that we were doing so, at least with high probability. I will give an example of the insights we gained from such work in chapter 5.

Third, in certain kinds of Internet websites, people are more likely to be truthful. There are many examples of the opposite, but one of my favorites was detailed in a blog entry[29] at OKCupid.com, an online dating site. According to measurements from that website, people tend to exaggerate their height by 2 inches, overstate their income by 20 percent, and misstate their sexual preferences. For example, 80 percent of self-identified bisexuals are in fact interested in only one gender. There is a good reason to lie about things such as income: Low-income men over the age of 23 are unlikely to get any messages from females. (Younger males are allowed to be poor, apparently.) When people have a good reason to lie, they lie. However, this incentive disappears when people are anonymous, as, for example, when they query a search engine or go to anonymous social forums such as Yahoo Answers.

We cannot verify that each and every user is truthful, because we cannot go and ask them (or go over their medical file). However, we can compare averages of the entire population. When we do that, we find that the number of people who ask about the specific types of cancer, such as thyroid cancer, is highly correlated with the incidence of these diseases reported by the United States' Centers for Disease Control. Similarly, the number of people querying for a certain drug is highly correlated with the number of prescriptions sold for that drug.

Fourth, when the activity we want to learn about takes place on the Internet, that's the best place to learn about it. Some diseases are relatively rare, striking, say, one person in 100,000. Before the Internet, people with such diseases had difficulty finding one another. Today, however, the Internet serves as a virtual meeting place for them, providing advice, support, and solace.

Some of the meeting places for people with rare diseases are truly remarkable, and few are as remarkable as PatientsLikeMe. com. Stephan Heywood, a self-taught architect and builder, was diagnosed with Amyotrophic Lateral Sclerosis (ALS) at the age of 29. ALS is a rare disease that causes motor neurons (the nerve cells that command muscles to move) to degenerate until the patient dies, often from the inability to breathe. There is no known cure for the disease. Stephan died eight years after he was first diagnosed, but his brothers and a family friend founded PatientsLikeMe, a site at which people with ALS can find other people with the disease and share their questions and experiences with them.

Not long after it was founded, PatientsLikeMe became a popular meeting place for people with other rare diseases, and even for people with more common chronic diseases. Today it serves more than 200,000 patients suffering from 1,500 diseases. Significantly, it is the largest community for ALS patients on the Internet. On the website, people report their medical conditions, sometimes at a very fine level of detail, but also ask some rather mundane questions. While PatientsLikeMe has surely helped patients, it has also helped advance medical research by drawing on the experiences of those patients. For example, a small clinical study suggested that lithium carbonate can delay the progression of ALS. By comparing patients on PatientsLikeMe who reported taking this supplement with those who did not, Paul Wicks and his colleagues showed that lithium carbonate was not, in fact, useful for that purpose.[30]

Similar websites, and ad hoc communities, exist for many patient groups. Some patient groups, however, have a less savory aspect to them. A colleague once described to me a website he built for people suffering from anorexia. Soon after the site became active, he had to shut down its social networking feature because people were using it to share information on how to lose weight, not how to recover from their disease.

Websites that promote harmful practices are, unfortunately, abundant, especially for mental diseases. Later in this book I will describe sites that treat anorexia nervosa as a "lifestyle choice" and help visitors to hide their anorexia from family members and friends, to starve themselves and to find inspiring photographs of other emaciated people.

In all these cases, information generated online is the most pertinent information to study. I will describe several such websites, and what we learned from them, in the following chapters. However, before I delve into what we can learn from this content, I want to deal with a pertinent question that we tend to overlook: Why do people go to the Web for medical information in the first place? Wouldn't one's family doctor be the more appropriate person to ask? The next chapter describes our attempts to answer this question and to gain insights into where we should look for interesting medical information (and where we should not look); it also takes up the question of what kinds of data we can expect to find.

2   Answering the Unaskable

Dr. Franz Ingelfinger, a gastroenterologist and a former editor of the New England Journal of Medicine, *was diagnosed with cancer. In a 1980 lecture delivered after his diagnosis,*[1] *Dr. Ingelfinger described the distress caused by the flood of information aimed at him and his family. He praised one of his friends for telling him: "Forget the information you got from many quarters and look for a person who would simply tell you what to do. You need a doctor."*

Why do people use the Internet to ask medical questions? At first, it seems obvious that they ask because that's where the information is. But on second thought it is not so simple. The Web is notorious for providing misleading knowledge, it may overload a person with information, and most people have an obvious candidate for someone to answer their questions: their doctor. Moreover, if one's question is not anonymous, one may divulge potentially embarrassing information to friends and peers. This chapter addresses the question of why people use the Internet to ask medical questions. It also investigates a highly related question: Do they find what they are looking for?

The question of why people use the Internet for medical needs probably has as many answers as Internet users, so I will try to answer the question by making generalizations, hoping that my generalizations will not be too broad.

It is worth repeating that, according to Pew surveys, 85 percent of the adult population of the United States uses the Internet, and of those at least 80 percent use the Internet to address medical concerns. Therefore, seeking medical information is a relatively common online activity.

How knowing who you are affects what you can ask

One way to understand why the Internet is used for medical questions is to look at where medical information is sought. People can, and do, ask medical questions on a variety of sites. Dan Pelleg, Yoelle Maarek, and I compared four sites that are used to ask general questions and also to ask medically related questions.[2] We looked at postings on Facebook, Twitter, Google Groups (a site for topic-specific discussions) and Yahoo Answers (where users can ask questions which are then answered by other users). One important difference among these sites is how identifiable a person is—that is, how easy it is to identify a user and how easy it is to link a user's virtual persona to a person in the physical world.

If you live in an industrialized country, or if you have a landline telephone almost anywhere in the world, you probably have been surveyed for one reason or another. You receive a call, and at the other end of the line an eloquent young person identifies himself (or herself) and the company, makes sure that you are the person for whom the call is intended, and ask whether you are willing to answer a few questions. It will not take more than a few minutes of your precious time. Imagine yourself in that situation. Questions about what topics are you most likely to answer, and questions about what topics are you unlikely to answer? Remember that the caller identified you and thus knows who you are. Most people will (if they agree to be surveyed at all) answer questions about their favorite breakfast cereal or how long their commute is. But will you feel comfortable answering if the person asks what your monthly salary is, whether you browse the Internet for pornography, or what sort of porn you favor? Will you answer or will you hang up?

Telephone surveyors know that some topics are more difficult to get a truthful response for, especially if the survey is not anonymous—that is, if the surveyor knows who the subject is and the subject knows that the surveyor knows who he or she is. The most sensitive topics, at least in the Western world, are personal characteristics (e.g., weight and age), financial details (e.g., salary), and behaviors that might be socially sensitive (e.g., sexual behavior). When questions are on other topics, or when the answerer can remain anonymous, it is much easier to get a truthful response.

Dan, Yoelle, and I found similar behaviors online, especially with regard to medical questions. Medical questions can, of course, be sensitive. Will you feel comfortable graphically describing the results of that spoiled sushi you had last night to your friends, and asking whether you should see a doctor? Probably not. If you think you want to ask that question, you had better ask it where nobody knows who you are. Identifiability—the ability to know who you are in the real world, and to tie your virtual identity to your physical one—is important. Therefore, it is worth looking at how various popular websites grapple with identifiability.

Facebook's policy is that users must be identified in their real names. People on Twitter sometimes provide their real names, but more often they only give a pseudonym. However, because they are active for long periods of time, it is usually possible to identify them to some extent. Google Groups and Yahoo Answers are at the other extreme: They allow one to register with any user name one wishes to use, no matter how meaningless.

Posts on Facebook can be public (visible to anyone), or private (so that only friends can see them). And some Facebook postings are public for a while but are later removed from public view, either because the user who posted them decided he or she did not want to share the information or because the user decided to share the information with friends and make it private. It is illuminating to see what users removed once they had a second thought.

Private messages passed between friends tend to be about food, fun, and time. Many of them concern dinners, movies, and other leisure activities. When we compared public posts and posts that are later deleted, we found that there was a good reason to remove certain posts. They contained lots of profanity and information on digestion and other bodily activities. Therefore, it seems that people remove some posts to maintain a respectable public persona. Facebook users are aware of social norms and of their public image, as is evident from the fact that they later amend profanity, angry words, and mentions of sexual topics in their posts. Moreover, topics that are known to be sensitive, such as financial information, health-related data, and socially stigmatized activities, are virtually absent from Facebook. On Twitter, more of these sensitive topics are discussed. Indeed, some patient groups hold virtual "meetings" on Twitter.[3] Since Twitter is, to some extent, anonymous, even diseases that are stigmatized, such as mood disorders and various forms of addiction, can be discussed relatively freely. Although we did not test this, one can confidently guess that on Twitter, people who discuss sensitive topics will be closer to the more anonymous part of the spectrum than people who do not discuss sensitive topics.

Where anonymity rules, as it does on Yahoo Answers and Google Groups, so does sensitive information. When I became aware that at least 66,000 people used Yahoo Answers to ask questions such as "What should be helpful tips for 1st time intercourse?" I understood that I was probably of a different generation. We know that such topics are considered to be sensitive because people who conduct surveys have studied what topics people tend to lie about when they are asked about them in surveys. But on Yahoo Answers one can find about 80,000 questions of the form "I'm a 17 year-old male, 175 cm tall, 75 kg in weight. Am I fat?" In these questions users specify their age, their gender, their height, and their weight and ask "Am I fat?"[4] (or thin, obese, or underweight). Other questions, especially about taxes, specify users' incomes, and still others state their sexual behaviors. More generally, questions about health, relationships, sexuality, and actions that may or may not be legal are abundant on Yahoo Answers and Google Groups.

Interestingly, some users of Yahoo Answers reveal that they know their questions are sensitive. We observed a set of questions (which we dubbed the "secret questions") in which users will say "I can't talk to my parents about this" and ask the whole world to provide anonymous opinions about their problem. For example, one user asked "Do I Have A STD?!!!?!?!?!?!?!? I think I might have a STD I'm 14 and I can't tell my parents." Some of these questions are heartbreaking, and others may be silly, but they represent a need for knowledge that only anonymous venues such as Yahoo Answers can address. Some people, unfortunately, feel that they cannot ask such questions of their friends, other members of their social circle, or family members. Many parents are "friends" of their children on Facebook, and posting the question on such an identifiable website would immediately lead to a stern talk at the dinner table. On Yahoo Answers, where one can be anonymous, parents will be none the wiser.

"Secret questions" tell us what is hidden and who it is hidden from. Relationship problems are often hidden from spouses, but also from close friends. Interestingly, we found that there were many problems that a female asker said she could not discuss with her boyfriend, but virtually none that a male asker said he could not discuss with his girlfriend. This does not mean that men have fewer problems, only that they are less likely to discuss them. Similarly, financial issues, family problems, health conditions, and sexual difficulties are not to be discussed with spouses. In all these cases, partners find it hard to communicate effectively with their loved ones. More troubling is the fact that askers are disinclined to discuss problems with teachers, perhaps because they view them as outsiders. And some askers feel that they cannot discuss medical problems, including matters of diet, physical health, and mental health, with medical doctors. Whether this is because people feel that they know their doctors too well or not well enough, the result is the same. The possibility that they think they do not know their doctors well enough is supported by evidence that patients do not disclose the information they have to their doctors for fear that they will be stigmatized.[5] For example, a cancer patient who is considering turning to alternative medicine for additional treatment may fear that his doctor will try to dissuade him or will later think less of him. For all such matters, the anonymous venue of Yahoo Answers is a good outlet.

Users, however, are not satisfied with the ability to ask anonymous questions on Yahoo Answers, and take additional steps to hide their tracks. One group of users maintains two online personas. One is used to interact with the community, to ask non-sensitive questions, and to answer other users' questions; the other is used only to ask sensitive questions. Other users hide some of their personal details when asking sensitive questions, or provide fake details. And some users simply delete their sensitive questions once they have received sufficient answers.

Clearly, users are aware that they are exposing a sensitive part of their world. What do they gain from doing so? First, many of the responses they obtain are thoughtful and accurate. Although as questions become more elaborate the accuracy of the answers decreases, many of the questions concern minor medical issues and receive precise answers. Askers who mark some of the responses as the best answers they receive have a very slight (under 1 percent) preference for the answers that have a higher informational content, but have a clear preference for answers that provide emotional support (a 6 percent increase in questions chosen as "best"). Much of the information people seek on Yahoo Answers can be found by querying a search engine such as Google or Bing; however, people seeking emotional support and more sensitive information go directly to Yahoo Answers.

When people provide an answer on Yahoo Answers they gain points. Even though these points are good for almost nothing except raising a user's ranking on the site, people like getting them. This is probably why, even when people ask questions that are likely to draw cheap shots in talkback on news sites, they receive courteous answers on Yahoo Answer. For example, one user asked "I am a 5'5 female, and weight 94 kg, am I obese?" According to the guidelines issued by the U.S. Centers for Disease Control, she is clearly obese, and she would be easy to answer in a denigrating way. Instead, she received a more considerate reply, which began: "Well, unfortunately you are extremely overweight. It's a sad situation but you need to do something about it."

The point here is that people use Yahoo Answers to seek medical information that often is sensitive and so cannot be asked in a forum where people know them. They do, however, want the personal touch.

Search engines provide an anonymous venue for medical queries and thus offer a service similar to that offered by Yahoo Answers, albeit without the emotional support or the personal touch. The advantage of search engines lies in their immediacy, which is hard for more "social" websites to beat. Thus, it is not surprising that when we measure the correlation between the number of questions about aspects of real life behavior and their known frequency in the world, for example, the correlation between the incidence of disease and the number of people asking about it on Bing, it correlates very well with measurements from the real world.

In a similar vein, medical forums provide both emotional support and medical information, but not anonymity. This is especially true at websites where users post information over long periods of time, such as patientslikeme.com and other patient forums.

Availability of access and ease of use also influence why people choose the Internet as a source for medical information, above and beyond anonymity. First, many people lack access to medical care. Before the Affordable Care Act ("Obamacare"), 49.9 million people in the United States,[6] or 16.3 percent of the population, did not have health insurance. It is still difficult to obtain good data for the number of uninsured people after the implementation of the Affordable Care Act, but it is safe to assume that some people still do not have health insurance and consequently find it difficult to gain access to medical care. Moreover, it is estimated that 21 percent of adults with health insurance in the United States are underinsured, meaning that they usually have to pay significant amounts of money to seek care.[7] As a result, when a medical problem appears, they can choose to go to the emergency room of a local hospital or try to find a solution to their woes online. This was apparent when we looked at the queries people make on search engines upon learning that they or a close relative have been diagnosed with cancer. One of the terms that appear most often in queries in conjunction with different types of cancers is "free." An oncologist suggested that this might be referring to "disease free survival," but when we looked at the queries closely it became apparent that the context was "free diagnosis" and "free treatment," probably because the people who submitted the queries had no other option for obtaining treatment.

Even though access to medical providers is available to the majority of people in industrialized countries, immediate access may not be easy to obtain, especially when specialists are involved. It can also be costly or require lengthy travel. Therefore, people often prefer to perform an initial screening of their problem online. (Is that wart something that needs immediate medical attention, or can it wait two weeks for my yearly checkup? What are my chances of pregnancy after last night's escapades?)

Interestingly, such screening (or self-diagnosis) is evident even for life-threatening conditions. Ryen White and Eric Horvitz documented the time it takes from when a person issues a query on a specific symptom till the person tries to find a medical facility for its treatment.[8] Abdominal pain, headaches, dizziness, and chest pain all lead to a medical facility in under 5 hours. In comparison, it takes between 20 and 30 hours before a person who queried for nausea, joint pain, or back pain seeks a medical provider. Interestingly, even when people query for chest pain, one of the important indications for a heart attack, it takes them about 3 hours before they decide to find a hospital, instead of taking immediate action. However, it may be that most people who query for chest pain recognize the danger they may be in and, instead of staying at their computer, make a telephone request for emergency care.

Therefore, the answer to why people go to the Internet for medical information is a complicated mix of several factors, including privacy, accuracy of information, speed of access, and emotional support.

Is medical information available online useful to those who seek it?

By the standards cited above, do people find the information and the support they were looking for? The scientific literature is divided on that question. On the one hand, the Pew Research Center's Internet & American Life Project[9] reports that, in surveys, 41 percent of people who made a diagnosis of their condition from online data said that the diagnosis was confirmed by their doctor, whereas only 18 percent who reported that their doctor disagreed. Most of the remaining people did not go to a doctor, so one can only guess whether their diagnosis was correct.

On the other hand, a large number of papers purport to show that online medical information is grossly inaccurate. For example, some groups who oppose vaccines still claim that the Mumps-Measles-Rubella vaccine causes autism, even though the study that originally made that link was retracted and the claim was refuted by multiple follow-up studies. Others peddle alternative medicine as the sole treatment for cancer.

Some websites err on the side of caution, providing information on all the options even if these options are extremely rare and unlikely. This leads many people to what's been called Cyberchondria.[10] White and Horvitz defined cyberchondria as when someone suffering from what is very likely to be a completely innocuous (though perhaps uncomfortable) symptom, searches the Web for information about it, and then comes to think he or she has a much more serious condition. This can happen, for example, when I search for "headache" and decide that I have a brain tumor, or that I have a muscle twitch which then leads me to think I am suffering from ALS, a fatal neurological disease.

Cyberchondria is only a manifestation of the older phenomena of hypochondria, so beautifully summarized in Jerome K. Jerome's 1889 book *Three Men in a Boat.*[11] Allow me to quote from that remarkable book:

I remember going to the British Museum one day to read up the treatment for some slight ailment of which I had a touch—hay fever, I fancy it was. I got down the book, and read all I came to read; and then, in an unthinking moment, I idly turned the leaves, and began to indolently study diseases, generally. I forget which was the first distemper I plunged into—some fearful, devastating scourge, I know—and, before I had glanced half down the list of "premonitory symptoms," it was borne in upon me that I had fairly got it.

I sat for a while, frozen with horror; and then, in the listlessness of despair, I again turned over the pages. I came to typhoid fever—read the symptoms—discovered that I had typhoid fever, must have had it for months without knowing it—wondered what else I had got; turned up St. Vitus's Dance—found, as I expected, that I had that too,—began to get interested in my case, and determined to sift it to the bottom, and so started alphabetically—read up ague, and learnt that I was sickening for it, and that the acute stage would commence in about another fortnight. Bright's disease, I was relieved to find, I had only in a modified form, and, so far as that was concerned, I might live for years. Cholera I had, with severe complications; and diphtheria I seemed to have been born with. I plodded conscientiously through the twenty-six letters, and the only malady I could conclude I had not got was housemaid's knee.

I felt rather hurt about this at first; it seemed somehow to be a sort of slight. Why hadn't I got housemaid's knee? Why this invidious reservation? After a while, however, less grasping feelings prevailed. I reflected that I had every other known malady in the pharmacology, and I grew less selfish, and determined to do without housemaid's knee. Gout, in its most malignant stage, it would appear, had seized me without my being aware of it; and zymosis I had evidently been suffering with from boyhood. There were no more diseases after zymosis, so I concluded there was nothing else the matter with me.

I sat and pondered. I thought what an interesting case I must be from a medical point of view, what an acquisition I should be to a class! Students would have no need to "walk the hospitals," if they had me. I was a hospital in myself. All they need do would be to walk round me, and, after that, take their diploma.

In an attempt to deal with inaccuracies of medical information, a non-profit organization called Health On The Net certifies websites for the reliability and usefulness of the medical information they display. However, only about 5,000 websites are currently certified, whereas about 49,000 health-related websites are listed in the manually curated Open Directory Project. Moreover, because the certification is completely voluntary, very little can be done about websites that do not live up to Health On The Net's standard. Thus, although people report finding good medical information on the Web, the data tell a more nuanced story.

How accurate are the data people provide about themselves?

Because people feel that some of the information they provide is sensitive, it is worthwhile to test how much this information can tell us about these people and how accurate the information is. Although we cannot evaluate the accuracy of each bit of information, we can check whether, on average, the information is accurate. As we have seen, several real-world behaviors (e.g., prescriptions filled and the incidence of cancer) correlate well with the frequency of queries about these behaviors in search-engine logs. Let me give a few more examples from Yahoo Answers.

Whenever a user of Yahoo Answers asks a question, that user is asked to catalog the question into one of approximately 1,700 categories. The categories include, for example, homework, travel, and pregnancy. Figure 2.1 shows a small part of a larger chart that was constructed by measuring the average number of months between questions in one category and questions in another. For example, a person who asked a question in the Pregnancy category will typically ask a question in the Newborn and Baby category after 8 months. After another 15 months, the person is likely to ask a question in the Toddler category.

On average, 18 months pass between when someone asks a dating-related question and when that person asks about pregnancy. This is the same amount of time required for dealing with

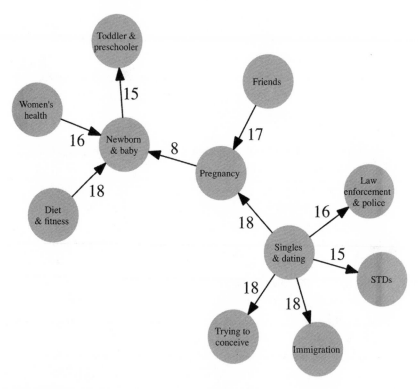

Figure 2.1
The average number of months between questions in different categories
on Yahoo Answers.

immigration issues if one's spouse is not from one's own country or (if pregnancy has not occurred naturally) inquiring in the Trying to Conceive category. Incidentally, those anxious would-be parents who ask questions in the Trying to Conceive category need only wait another two weeks, by which time they would typically start asking in the Pregnancy category. Sexually transmitted diseases (STDs) take less time to surface, characteristically appearing 15 months after the start of dating. And 16 months is, on average, how long it takes for a relationship to sour to the extent that the police are needed to remove one partner from the home, as one can see by looking at the questions in the category "Law Enforcement and Police."

These transitions are an anecdotal demonstration of a much more serious phenomenon. We know from personal experience that at least some of the transitions mentioned above are meaningful—for example, the typical gestation period is 9 months. Thus, users are revealing their real behavior by posting their questions. Moreover, I predict that, were someone to consider all the questions of a single user who likes to ask about each and every problem he or she has, it would not be overly difficult to identify that individual in the real world, just as the AOL log helped to reveal Thelma Arnold's identity. Therefore, users do well when they take steps to anonymize their questions, at least those that pertain to the more sensitive aspects of their lives.

As I mentioned in the preceding chapter, many people ask about what they know are sensitive social behaviors, of which one of the most common is teenage sexual intercourse. A common question begins "Tips for first time sex? I am 15 and my boyfriend of a year and a half is 17." Here we are given the age of first intercourse (which the Centers for Disease Control also

measures through surveys, the latest being from 2002[12]) of teen-
agers and young adults. When we compared the age at which
people asked about first time intercourse against the ages
reported in Kinsey Institute surveys, we found an almost perfect
match. The main differences were that Kinsey did not interview
people under the age of 15, whereas Yahoo Answers shows questions by people as young as 13, and that Kinsey did not interview people over the age of 24, though quite a few people ask for
such advice but report being over 24.

Another demonstration of the accuracy of information provided in questions lies in the 80,000 or so questions in which
users specify their age, gender, height, and weight and then ask
"Am I fat?" (or thin, or obese, or underweight). Comparing the
average weight and height reported by age and gender shows a
very good match between these questions and measurements of
teenagers conducted by the CDC. The details are, though, more
interesting than the average. Men, it turns out, estimate their
weight fairly well: When a man asks "Am I underweight?" he
usually is. Similarly, men who ask "Am I fat?" or "am I obese?"
usually are, in fact, overweight or clinically obese. Women are
not as good at estimating their weight: Women who ask "Am I
underweight?" or "Am I obese?" correctly recognize that they
are on one or the other end of the weight spectrum. Women
who ask "Am I fat?" are, in line with the stereotype, slightly
below the median weight reported by the CDC.

Consequently, people are right to assume that the information they provide when asking any question, and especially
when asking a sensitive question, reveals aspects of their life that
might contribute to a breach of their privacy, and to assume that
such a breach might reveal important and perhaps unsavory
information about them. From the point of view of a researcher,

however, these data, when used in what I believe is a privacy-preserving manner, represent a boon to scientific inquiry.

Much as Professor Ingelfinger found the information flowing from well-intentioned people to be overwhelming, it seems that nowadays, even though information on the Internet is more abundant than it was in Ingelfinger's day, it allows people to target their searches and to receive more specific information. More important, perhaps, it enables people to receive emotional support from like-minded individuals or, at least, individuals in similar situations. Today, Professor Ingelfinger's friend might have told him "You need a doctor, and a good online support group."

3 Anorexia: A Disease Online

In the course of one of my studies on eating disorders, I used photographs that people had posted on a photo-sharing site to characterize those individuals' stances with regard to anorexia. I browsed the images (mostly of emaciated women) and decided, on the basis of those images and the accompanying text, whether the individuals in question were for or against eating disorders. One of my colleagues passed my cubicle, saw the images I was labeling, and remarked "Good thing you only have boys."

In earlier chapters we saw that some conditions should be studied using Internet data because the Internet is where much of the activity of patients takes place. Before the Internet, people with relatively rare diseases had difficulty finding one another. Today the Internet serves as a virtual meeting place for these people, providing advice on recovery, but also, astoundingly, on how to become sicker. This is especially true for certain mental diseases, such as anorexia. In this chapter I describe what we learned about anorexia from what patients say about it online. These lessons, which would have been difficult to learn in any other way, taught us about the harmful effects of good intentions. They also showed how words used to describe a celebrity can cause real harm.

Anorexia nervosa is a terrible disease. Defined as a mental disorder in the American Psychiatric Association's *Diagnostic and Statistical Manual of Mental Health Disorders* (DSM), the latest version of which is DSM-5, anorexia nervosa is characterized by a fear of gaining weight, and leading consequently, to self-starvation. Estimates are that anorexia nervosa kills between 2 percent and 14 percent of sufferers, who are predominantly young women, and even those who recover from the disease rarely experience complete recovery.

Strictly speaking, anorexia is a lack of appetite, but colloquially anorexia usually refers to the mental disorder anorexia nervosa. Hence, here I will use the shortened term. Another problem of terminology is that anorexia nervosa literally means a neurotic loss of appetite. However, research has found that this is not the case in many patients of anorexia. Indeed, these people are very hungry (even their hormone levels tell us this), but have decided to starve themselves in an attempt to improve a distorted image of themselves.

Starving oneself is difficult. The body repeatedly tries to signal the brain that it needs food, and overriding this urge requires an anorexic to work hard. There was a time when each anorexic had to do this by herself, but today there are many websites devoted to helping people starve, which is how we know it is hard. For example, at one site devoted to anorexia, in a discussion of the merits of eating a single meal per day, a user wrote: "I eat a small meal at the end of my day, so I can get to sleep. I have a hard time sleeping hungry."[1]

Pro-anorexia content: "a lifestyle, not a disease"

Before the advent of the Internet, an anorexia sufferer was unlikely to meet a like-minded individual, except perhaps at a clinic for eating-disorder patients. With a prevalence ranging from 1 percent to 4 percent, it would have been rare to meet another person with the disease and share information with her. The Internet changed all that. By a conservative estimate there now are at least 600 sites[2] dedicated solely to encouraging disordered eating, and many mainstream websites (e.g., photosharing sites such as Flickr) contain pro-anorexia content. These websites cater to a community known as "pro-anorexia," "pro-ana," or simply "ana."

At these sites, anorexia is not a disease. Indeed, the motto of one site is "Anorexia is a lifestyle, not a disease."[3] Other sites have more nuanced stances, claiming, for example, to "support the recovery of the individual when they are ready."[4] However, scratch the surface and you will find that site operators and participants show indifference to, and more often encouragement of, disordered eating, often by people who are experiencing it themselves.

Websites that cater to anorexia patients provide various kinds of support. Some provide collections of photographs designed in encourage weight loss, some give information to help starve oneself, and some provide social support.

Sites in the first category, known colloquially as "thinspiration" sites, include photos of celebrities who are known to be, or suspected of being, anorexic, mostly photographed in ways that emphasize their skeleton-like features, and of anorexia patients bragging of their weight loss by showing their current appearance. Not surprisingly, most of these photographs focus on the stomach, the collarbone, and the thighs.

Sites in the second category provide information on dieting and on how to deal with one's family. Since starving is hard, anorexia patients have developed a range of diets. One, the so-called 2468 diet, encourages people to consume 200 calories on the first day, 400 calories on the second day, 600 calories on the third day, 800 calories on the fourth day, fast on the fifth day, and then repeat. For comparison, the recommended daily caloric intake for a woman is 2,000 calories.[5] Prisoners at Auschwitz received between 1,300 and 1,700 calories a day; the upper range, though grossly insufficient, was reserved for those who performed hard manual labor.[6]

Once they become aware that something is wrong, most parents of minors with an eating disorder try to help their ailing children by making sure they eat. Therefore, many websites for anorexics provide advice on how to mislead one's parents into thinking all is well. Some of the advice is banal ("Wake up late, so you don't have enough time to eat at home"[7]; "Say you've already ate"); some is more elaborate. One plan suggests five tactics: Ask questions to divert your parents' attention away from your food. Talk a lot. Spit food into a napkin. Make the amount of food you have not eaten look smaller by pushing it to one part of the plate. Offer other people some of your food.[8]

Perhaps most important, pro-anorexia websites provide help in finding support. Some of the support is in the form of forums in which anorexics can rant about their parents, siblings, and friends to like-minded people. Other sites help people with eating disorders find "pro-ana buddies" who will help them to maintain their disordered behaviors. A typical request reads "I am looking for a SERIOUS pro ana buddy. Someone I can call and text whenever I feel cravings. I am seriously overweight, and need to lose it FAST. I love the pro ana community. I want a pro ana buddy who has been anorexic for a while and someone who is dedicated."[9]

These websites are quite effective in what they purport to do. Examples of their harm abound in the media. Grainne Binns, an

Irish teenager, claims to have become addicted to posting pictures of her skeletal frame on "thinspiration" sites and to checking comments that her virtual "friends" left.[10] Studies have shown that young women are very aware of pro-anorexia sites: According to one study, at least 12 percent of young teenage women in Belgium reported viewing pro-anorexia content. Perhaps more worrying, studies have shown that viewing of pro-anorexia content is correlated with worsening of anorexia.

The media connection to anorexia

In view of the difficulty people experience when attempting to become anorexic, one has to wonder what triggers the disease. Anorexia usually starts in adolescence, and more frequently in girls than in boys. Alarmingly, the age range of onset for anorexia has been decreasing over the past few years, from 13–17 years down to 9–12. We know of many factors that put people in risk of developing anorexia, or that occur in conjunction with it. A need for self-control, an inclination toward perfectionism, anxiety, and depression all put people at risk of developing anorexia.

Some people have suggested that external factors are also to blame. One suspect is the fashion industry. "Fifteen to 20 years ago, we shot models [in the European clothing size] 38. Today it's 24," said Adi Barkan, an Israeli fashion photographer. "This is the difference between thin and too thin. This is the difference between death and life."[11] The logic of the thin-models argument is that fashion models are role models for young women, who see them as exemplars of society's beauty ideal. These models are widely published and shown in the media, thus encouraging anorexia and other eating disorders. But this hypothesis is hard to measure in the physical world. In order to test it in the real world, one would have to choose a large population of people, expose some of them to underweight models and some of them to models of normal weight, and see whether, after weeks or months of such exposure, more members of the first group develop anorexia. It is, of course, not realistic to perform such an experiment, except perhaps in a controlled world such as that depicted in the movie *The Truman Show* or in a world in which a large enough percentage of people are wearing Google Glasses (which can continuously photograph everything ta wearer is seeing). In the virtual world, however, such measurements are not very difficult.[12] Whenever a person searches for a celebrity or a model, the search-engine company logs the actual text of the search (e.g., "Angelina Jolie"), what images and links were shown to the user by the search engine, and which of those links the user clicked on. This allows us to measure exposure to celebrities over a period of months.

But how do we know if people search for a celebrity because of the person's celebrity status, or because the celebrity is anorexic, or even because the celebrity is widely thought to be anorexic? To do this we devised a score we called the Perceived Anorexia Score—a fancy name for the likelihood that the word "anorexia" will appear in conjunction with a celebrity's name whenever that person's name is queried. It is a simple measure, but it is quite effective: 32 percent of the celebrities with the highest Perceived Anorexia Scores admitted publicly to suffering from anorexia, and a further 49 percent were rumored to suffer from it.

That leaves one final problem before we can measure whether there is an association between exposure to anorexic celebrities and the development of anorexia: How can we determine which of the people who used search engines to query the names of anorexic celebrities have anorexia themselves?

The surest way would have been to contact each of them and ask. Both for reasons of scale (we looked at the activity of about 9 million people) and because of concerns about privacy, that was not feasible. Instead, we looked for the typical queries of people who frequent pro-anorexia websites, and found that their queries fell into three major categories: queries for tips for people with anorexia (e.g., "tips for anorexia"), do-it-yourself queries (e.g., "how to become anorexic?"), and queries intended to help find pro-anorexia "buddies" (i.e., people who will help the sufferer maintain their condition and lose more weight). That someone posts such queries does not tell us that she has a clinical diagnosis of anorexia, but it is a strong indication for it.

Armed with this knowledge, we looked at five months of queries submitted to all major search engines by a population of about 9 million people. We chose these people because they queried at least once for a celebrity with a high Perceived Anorexia Score. Of those 9 million people, 2,060 later made queries that we classified as typical of an anorexic.

Many areas of medicine and insurance ask how likely a person is to survive for the next few days, months, or years in view of his or her circumstances. If data from a large enough population can be gathered, we can plot a graph that answers this question. For example, if we take a large population of women who have been diagnosed with breast cancer and wait a sufficiently long period, we can plot a graph that will show the likelihood that a women will survive for a month, a year, or a decade after the initial diagnosis simply by counting how many women survived for these periods in our cohort of patients. Such a graph is known as a *survival curve*.

A more specific question that is of interest to medical practitioners is, in many cases, slightly different from the one that is answered by a survival curve. It is instead: Given that a patient has survived thus far, what is the likelihood that the patient will die, or suffer a recurrence of the illness, in the next day, week, or month? This likelihood, which is technically computed as the ratio between the probability of recurrence in the next time period and the same probability up to now, is known as the *hazard function*. The hazard function can be interesting by itself if we want to estimate recurring diseases or recurring visits to hospitals. But there are more fascinating uses for it.

In 1972, D. R. Cox showed how to estimate the contributions of various variables to the hazard. This enabled epidemiologists to ask, for example, whether the ages of women diagnosed with breast cancer were associated with a higher or a lower hazard. More important, Cox's method enabled us to use data observed only over a limited time period. After Cox's paper was presented to the Royal Statistical Society, a researcher from Oxford University remarked that his method "opened up new territories to common sense."[13]

Our common-sense measurement was to estimate the increase or decrease in hazard of asking one of the typical anorexia queries (and hence, possibly suffering from anorexia) given a number of factors related to viewing celebrity content. For example, is there an elevated hazard to asking an anorexia query for users who use search engines a lot? The answer that came back was a definite No. There is no elevation or reduction of risk. The same is true for those people who are generally interested in celebrities. However, searching for a celebrity with a high anorexia score carries a significant hazard, and searching for more than one such celebrity increases this hazard by a factor of 9. This seemed a very definite finding: Apparently, viewing celebrities who are perceived as anorexic is correlated with later making queries that are typical of an anorexic. However, it still does not prove that one induces the other. Perhaps our users were already on the path to becoming anorexic, and viewing this content was just a precursor signal that anorexia was coming.

Worse, when danah boyd, a researcher at Microsoft, and I examined who the celebrities most often perceived as anorexic were, we discovered a troubling finding: Although many of them were indeed known or suspected to be suffering from anorexia, some of them had recovered from the disease and others were long dead. The question this raises is "Why would anyone, let alone a large number of people, suddenly be interested in a deceased celebrity?"

Answers to both of the questions mentioned above came from Twitter. It has been known for a few years that Twitter, the popular microblogging service that limits entries to 140 characters, is a good reflection of happenings in the mainstream media. One reason for this is that most mainstream media companies tweet their news. The other reason, stemming from the first, is that people who follow these media companies re-tweet news items that are interesting to them, and their followers repeat the process, thus creating a wave of tweets of news items that interest many people.

We tried to see how mentions of celebrities on Twitter correlated with searches people made using search engines. First, we saw that most searches and most mentions of a celebrity on Twitter tend to look like a wave, peaking almost at the same time. Interestingly, the sizes of the waves were highly correlated: The more Tweets about a celebrity, the more searches came later. This implies that the trigger for searches about celebrities in general, and those perceived as anorexic in particular, is media attention. When an article is written or a news story is shown about these celebrities, information about it is broadcast on Twitter. This article also causes people to go to their favorite search engine and search for more information about the celebrity. This explains why we saw interest in celebrities who were already out of the public eye: A journalist may have mentioned them in their reports, and that may have increased interest in them in the public arena.

The story, however, does not end there. We wanted to add these insights into our measures, but to distinguish between two ways in which a celebrity could be mentioned on Twitter: a way that is either appreciative or neutral and a way that mentions the celebrity's predicament. Therefore, we asked whether there is a hazard to the existence of a media wave on Twitter before people make their first anorexic query, and whether there is a different hazard when the media mention the word "anorexia" in their reporting during the wave.

At first our findings surprised us, but then they made complete sense. We found that there is a high hazard to the existence of a wave before an anorexic query, which indicates that these media waves do, in fact, drive later anorexic queries. However, when media reporting mentions anorexia, this hazard is almost completely removed, meaning that most people who would have begun to make anorexia queries will not do so.

The complete story is, then, that information on the Internet aids people in becoming anorexic. A major part of this information, and especially being aware to it, is driven by media reports about celebrities who are perceived as suffering from an eating disorder. Positive or indifferent reporting on those celebrities seems to cause people to develop anorexia. However, when these reports indicate that this celebrity is sick with anorexia, such a path does not appear, perhaps because people do not aspire to be sick—they want to be thin.

A similar phenomenon has been alleged for many years in regard to suicide. In 1774 Johann Wolfgang von Goethe published *The Sorrows of Young Werther*, a novel that describes a young man who decides to commit suicide after being rejected by the woman he loves. Soon after the novel's publication there were reports of young men using a method similar to that described by Goethe to kill themselves. This became known as the Werther Effect, and that term now is used to describe the phenomenon of when reporting about suicides leads to "copycat" suicides. In the words of David Shaffer, a professor of child psychiatry at Columbia University: "Hearing about a suicide moves those teen-agers at risk closer to doing it themselves."[14] The Werther Effect made the Centers for Disease Control recommended that newspapers never mention suicide in a headline and that news reports use the phrase "died by suicide" rather than "committed suicide," so as to emphasize the outcome and minimize any hint of empowerment.

We think there is a similar process at work with anorexia. When a celebrity is mentioned favorably as being very thin but beautiful, people at risk may develop anorexia because they perceive it as socially acceptable or even desirable. When a report frames anorexia in the opposite manner, few people want to follow an anorexic celebrity's example.

In Israel, a law bars the media from showing images of underweight models. Our findings suggest that that law is grounded in facts. On the Internet, however, it is easy to find content that is not subject to Israeli laws, and in the United States sites that tried to ban anorexic content[15] found it difficult to do so. Therefore, I think anorexia should be treated much as suicides are, and that news reports about anorexic celebrities should take care to say that they are sick with anorexia.

Harmful intervention

So far we have seen one path people take into anorexia. We have also wondered about the paths to help people recover from it. One of these taught us about the harmful effect of good intentions, and this is its story.

Flickr is a photo-sharing site run by Yahoo. It was started in 2004, and by 2011 had amassed more than 6 billion photographs from many tens of millions of users. Many of the pictures were taken by families on vacation, during day to day life, or by professional photographers hoping to sell their work. But over the years, more and more communities interested in certain themes have emerged within the site.

At the beginning of 2012 we noticed that the site hosted several hundreds of people who were using Flickr to share pro-anorexia ("thinspiration") photographs. These included the usual mix of photographs showing extremely thin celebrities and images taken by people themselves to show off their achievements in losing weight.

But, in addition to the pro-anorexia users, we[16] also found a sizable group of users who were posting content that emphasized the negative aspects of anorexia. Many of them had themselves suffered from the disease. After describing her disease and how she developed it, one of them wrote: "I'm done hurting my body. Starting now I'm going to love every inch of myself.

I'm going to get past everything that held me back and I'm going to help every girl I can to do the same."[17] Others were shocked by the damage the disease was doing, and decided to act. Many of them were posting photographs showing the bodily damage caused by anorexia and textual descriptions of its mental effects.

Flickr was especially interesting for us because of the different ways people could express their social connections with other users of the site. We identified four ways in which this can be done:

- A user can leave a comment on anyone's photograph. If the receiver of the comment is unhappy with it, she can delete the comment. Thus, a comment in place shows (to some extent) that the receiver was not terribly unhappy with it.

- It is possible to mark a Flickr user as a contact, but that user can remove the marking. Again, to a certain degree, because contact lists can be moderated, having a contact suggests that the user likes the contact, or at least does not dislike the person greatly.

- A user can mark a photograph as a favorite. In contrast with the previous two ways, the owner of a photograph marked as favorite by someone else cannot remove the marking.

- Users are encouraged to tag photographs when they upload them to Flickr. Since search engines do not understand the image in a way a human does, they rely on the text which accompanies photographs in order to find them when users search for images. For example, if a user adds the tag "winter" to a photograph, it increases the likelihood that this photo will appear in the results of another users' query for "winter" photos. If two users typically apply the same tags to their photographs, we can decide to mark them as connected, signifying that they have similar interests.

We could definitively identify 172 users as pro-recovery and 319 as pro-anorexia. About a fifth of the pro-recovery users stated in the text accompanying their photographs that they had recovered from, or were recovering from, anorexia or some other eating disorder.

As was described above, tags are a good way to typify a person or a group of persons. The tags most common in the pro-anorexia group and least common in the pro-recovery group were all related to anorexia, including those describing body parts ("legs," "body"), weight loss ("thinspiration," "skinny," "thin"), or positive images of women ("doll," "long," "model"). In contrast, the tags most common in the pro-recovery group, but least common in the pro-anorexia group, were a diverse mix, including "home," "sign," "selfportrait," "glass," and "sunshine." Thus, while the pro-recovery group seems to have a broad set of interests, the pro-anorexia group can be classified by their disease.

This could lead us to expect that by observing only tags one could easily identify pro-anorexia users. It turns out that this is not the case. Tags one might expect to be associated mostly with pro-anorexia users are widely used by pro-recovery people. For example, the tag "thinspiration" was used by 37 percent of the pro-anorexia users and, unexpectedly, by 7 percent of pro-recovery users. Even the tag "pro-anorexia" was used by 2 percent of the pro-anorexia users and the same percentage of pro-recovery people to tag their images. Analyzing the entire set of tags revealed a similar pattern: Pro-recovery users are, on average, more similar in their tags to pro-anorexia users than pro-anorexia users are among themselves. Moreover, when we decided that two people have the same outlook on anorexia if they use similar tags, we quickly discovered that we could not, in fact, predict the outlook of a person on the basis of that of his fellow users' tags.

At this point one might conclude that pro-recovery and pro-anorexia users cannot be distinguished on Flickr. But there remain other social connections that might be useful. Interestingly, contacts and comments make it easy to assess the opinion (pro-anorexia or pro-recovery) of a user on the basis of the opinions of his or her commenting peers. That is, if I am given the stance of all the people who have commented on someone's photo, I can quite confidently predict their stances on anorexia. Using a similar process for favorite markings, however, does not help in distinguishing between users.

Why are contacts and comments so indicative of like-minded people (at least for our narrow interest in anorexia), while favorites and tags are not? We suspect the answer lies both with the person who creates the link and the person to whom the link is made. Recall that comments and contacts are moderated by the user to whom the comments or contact request were made. That user can remove comments. Thus, users with a pro-recovery attitude can favor a pro-anorexia user's photo, and they can use the same tags as the pro-anorexia users, but when they make a comment to a pro-anorexia user, or ask such a user to become a contact, they are rebuffed by the pro-anorexia user.

There remains the question of why pro-recovery individuals and pro-anorexia individuals use similar tags. The reason for that, I think, goes back to the why pro-recovery users post their photographs in the first place. Recall a comment I quoted above, made by a pro-recovery user: "I'm going to help every girl I can to [love her body and recover]." Many of the pro-recovery users post their photos with the hope that they will be read by pro-anorexia users who then will see the error of their ways and begin to recover. The only way their tags will get noticed by pro-anorexia users is if they are similar to those searched for by pro-anorexia users. Thus, they masquerade as pro-anorexia users, and in a typical pro-anorexia search (e.g., for "thinspiration") we find many photos that were, in fact, taken by pro-recovery users.

Does posting the pro-recovery photographs help pro-anorexia users see the light? In medical terms, is it a useful intervention? Regrettably, our data show that it is counterproductive. Suppose that you are a pro-anorexia user, and that your photo receives a comment from a like-minded user. How likely are you to stop posting your pro-anorexia content, even if you continue posting images unrelated to anorexia on Flickr? We found that 61 percent of users stopped posting pro-anorexia content within 3 months after the comment. An identical percentage of pro-recovery users stopped posting pro-anorexia content after a comment from a pro-anorexia user. Seventy-one percent of pro-recovery users who got a comment from a user with a similar stance stopped posting pro-anorexia content. However, only 46 percent of pro-anorexia users who received a comment from a pro-recovery user stopped posting pro-anorexia photos.

To put it differently, a pro-anorexia user who gets a comment from a pro-recovery user will typically become more entrenched in her activities, and less likely to stop. More precise mathematical models bear this out. This pattern of behavior may not be surprising, in view of comments that pro-recovery users make to pro-anorexia users. A typical comment is "You need help. Call your psychiatrist right away and get help and eat a cheeseburger!!!"[18] With the zeal of a convert, pro-recovery users try to convince people with eating disorders to mend their ways.

What would be a good intervention? So far, researchers have found mostly negative answers to this question. Most of the interventions that were tried failed. As I mentioned above, banning content does not seem to work when there are so many other viable alternatives. But there is one hint of what could work. A few years ago, researchers in the Netherlands asked Internet service providers to show a warning label, similar to those on cigarette packets, whenever a user tried to access pro-anorexia content.[19] This relatively subtle intervention worked well enough to reduce the number of people viewing this harmful content.

Anorexia is an example of a disease that is exacerbated by the Internet. But since the Internet exacerbates the disease, we should use the Internet as a tool for recovery. We have some insights into what does not work. Now we need to find new interventions and to test them in order to help people recover from this devastating disease, and to prevent others from falling into this disease.

4   Questions of Public Health

Scientific reasoning is therefore at all levels an interaction between two episodes of thought – a dialogue between two voices, the one imaginative and the other critical; a dialogue, if you like, between the possible and the actual, between proposal and disposal, between conjecture and criticism, between what might be true and what is in fact the case

P. B. Medawar, "The Hope of Progress"

Epidemiological research is the cornerstone of public health, since it informs decision makers about the risk factors of various diseases. In many cases, an epidemiologist will begin by forming a hypothesis as to what might cause a medical condition, then laboriously collect data to support the hypothesis. This process is, to a large extent, limited by the imagination of researchers. If no one thought cigarettes caused cancer, perhaps no one would collect the necessary data to prove this link. Even when one does form a hypothesis, collecting enough data may take years. Mass production of cigarettes began in the late nineteenth century, but the first quantitative study on the harms of smoking was not published until 1929.[1]

In this chapter I describe how the data collected to improve search engines can also be used to improve public health, not only because they are useful for studies that are based on a hypothesis but also because they can be used to create new hypotheses. We will see how our algorithms can scour search-engine data to discover adverse effects of drugs, to identify possible risk factors for disease, and to rapidly alert health authorities when a music festival becomes a breeding ground for disease.

Using Internet data to monitor the safety of drugs

In July 1956, the German pharmaceutical firm Chemie Grunethal began selling Thalidomide, a new wonder drug intended to treat coughs, colds, and headaches and to serve as a mild sleeping pill.[2] Among its many advantages were that taking a lethal dose was nearly impossible and that the drug curbed morning sickness in pregnant women. Licensed to be sold over the counter in most European countries, Thalidomide was soon selling as many prescriptions as aspirin.[3]

But by 1960 reports were coming in of nerve damage in patients who had taken Thalidomide for prolonged periods. More disturbing, a German doctor, Dr. Lenz, and an Australian doctor, Dr. McBride, reported horrendous birth defects in babies whose mothers had taken Thalidomide. Babies were being born with shortened or absent limbs, deformed eyes, and deformed hearts, and many died shortly after birth. Health authorities banned Thalidomide in early 1962. It is estimated that by then more than 10,000 children had been affected by the drug.[4]

After its withdrawal, in a curious twist of fate, Thalidomide was found to be useful for treating two serious diseases: leprosy and multiple myeloma (a type of blood cancer). It is, however, tightly controlled when given to patients suffering from those diseases, to make sure that no new babies suffer from its side effects.

In the United States, the Food and Drug Administration refused to allow Thalidomide to be approved, requesting more clinical trials to show that Thalidomide would not affect a fetus in the womb. Frances Kelsey, the officer in charge of this refusal in the face of pressure from the manufacturer, was awarded the President's Award for Distinguished Federal Civilian Service by John F. Kennedy, and legislation to strengthen the FDA's role in drug approval was passed. The case of Thalidomide was one of the first major cases of adverse reactions' being discovered after a drug had been approved for sale. In the aftermath of its banning, several countries formed regulatory bodies to approve medicines.

Since Thalidomide, several drugs that had passed new, more rigorous testing regimens before approval have been found to have serious adverse effects. Cerivastatin, sold by Bayer as Lipobay, was withdrawn for causing death through rhabdomyolysis, a condition in which muscles disintegrate. Troglitazone, an anti-diabetic drug, was recalled for causing extensive liver damage. Rofecoxib, sold under the brand name Vioxx, was withdrawn by Merck, after more than 80 million people had taken it, because it had been found to cause heart attacks and strokes after being taken for long periods of time.

To understand how these medicines got to the market, and why they were withdrawn, it makes sense to go back to the beginning and consider how medical drugs are approved for use in most Western countries.

Suppose that you were to develop a new drug—one that you thought would cure someone's medical condition. After rigorous testing on human cells and on animals, your drug would be tested in a Phase 1 trial.[5] It would be given to a small number of healthy people just to test its safety. If the drug were to be deemed safe, you would then proceed to a Phase 2 trial, in which the drug would be given to several tens or a few hundreds of ill people. The purpose of a Phase 2 trial is to test a new drug's efficacy. If the drug seems effective, a Phase 3 trial is conducted— the drug is tested against the best currently available treatment, or, if no comparable treatment is available, against a placebo. Several thousands of people participate in the experiment. Some receive the new drug and some receive the best currently available treatment, and usually neither the patients nor the medical providers know who received what. At the end of the trial, the experimenters gather the results, consider whether they show that the new drug is useful, and, if the answer is positive, ask the FDA to convene a committee to decide whether the drug should be sold.

This process is rigorous and can take from six to ten years to complete. It has been blamed for the rising costs of new drugs and for the declining motivation of drug companies to develop new drugs. However, as may be obvious from its description, it cannot test several important aspects of drug usage. First, some drugs are taken for decades. Side effects that take decades to develop cannot be discovered by clinical trials that last, at most, several years. Second, many clinical trials try to focus on a specific treatment, and exclude anyone who already uses other treatments. This means that interactions between drugs are not investigated, and if there is an interaction it is not likely to be discovered through a Phase 3 trial. Rare events are another class of side effects that are hard to discover through clinical trials. If a drug kills one person in a million, even a medium-size trial involving several thousand people is unlikely to discover it, simply because the odds are that the rare event will not occur during the trial. Finally, there has been plenty of evidence that trials are not conducted on representative samples of the human race, instead recruiting either students from Western universities or people in countries where patients can be recruited more cheaply, such as India. If a drug is dangerous to a specific group of people, its danger will surface only when someone from this group begins taking the drug, usually long after it is in the market. For example, African Americans require higher doses of Warfarin[6] (a drug used in the prevention of blood clots) than members of other ethnic groups, so if tests did not include African-American participants, doctors might give African-American patients inappropriately low doses of the drug.

How, then, do drug companies and governments discover when drugs have adverse or even fatal side effects? The answer is so-called Phase 4 trials. These are a mix of clinical trials and reports by the public that are done after a drug is approved for sale, and indeed sometimes years after it has been in clinical use. The U.S. Food and Drug Administration, for example, runs the so-called FDA Adverse Event Reporting System[7] (abbreviated FAERS) by which members of the public and medical practitioners can report adverse effects of drugs. A similar system called VAERS is used for reporting on the adverse reactions to vaccines. That only a few million reports have been submitted to the FAERS is probably attributable to the fact that not many people know about it.

Several companies have tried to use the wisdom of the crowd to improve detection of adverse reactions. One example is ehealthme.com. When you first register at the site, you are asked to give your personal details and to state what medicines you take and what side effects you have experienced. By doing this, you are contributing to a database that links medicines, side effects, and the people who might be affected. The benefit to someone who takes these medicines is immediate: You can see a report of which side effects were experienced by more than 10 million people (at the time of writing) for the drug you are taking. It also has tremendous value for research, as it represents the actual experience of patients.

A different approach is taken by a site called Treato. Instead of asking people to contribute their experience, Treato mines discussion forums to extract patients' experiences from reports such as "I took drug X and it caused me headaches. Anyone else experienced this?" The benefit to patients is the ability to see what side effects they might experience.

However, FAERS, VAERS, ehealthme, and Treato all rely on a patient or a caregiver to make the association between a drug and the side effect. What happens if a side effect takes a long time to appear? We thought that in such cases it might be hazardous to depend on patients. For that reason, we looked for an alternative approach—one based on search-engine logs.

As has already been noted, there is a high correlation between the number of people who search for a drug on a search engine and the number of prescriptions written in the United States for that drug. This implies that many of the people who are prescribed a drug search for it online. (Granted, some of the searches are made by family members and medical caregivers, but for now we will assume that most searches are conducted by patients.)

Using this insight, Evgeniy Gabrilovich and I thought to look at the searches of people who queried for a medicine, and then see if these people later searched for side effects. If enough of them did, it would indicate a possible side effect.[8] That was the idea, but the devil, as the saying goes, is in the details.

First and foremost, there is the problem of language. Whereas drugs have only a few names, for example, the brand name and the scientific or generic name, people have a plethora of ways to describe their ailments. A headache might be described as a migraine, as a throbbing head, as a pounding head, or as cephalalgia. To evaluate the severity of the side effects of a drug correctly, we have to, somehow, take account of all the different terms people use for them.

Second, some symptoms may be seasonal. If we measure the number of mentions of a symptom before and after someone took a drug, and we do so during spring, we may notice lots of complaints of allergy-like symptoms in the people who queried for any drug, but allergy symptoms will also be common in people who did not mention the drug. We need to remove those symptoms.

People can help us in solving the first problem. Suppose you are looking for information about the causes of double vision. You put the words "causes of double vision" into the search engine of your choice, but the results are not what you are looking for. A closer inspection reveals that several of the results refer to double vision by its medical name, diplopia. You might, therefore, change your search to "causes of diplopia," for which the documents the search engine will show are more likely to include your results. If we see enough people going on this path, starting from "double vision" and ending in "diplopia," we can conclude that "double vision" and "diplopia" are synonyms. And that is exactly what we did. We collected all the searches that ended in the Wikipedia description of a medical symptom, then went back to see if the earlier searches repeated themselves in many

users. This helped us to generate a dictionary of medical symptoms and their synonyms as a layperson would describe them.

We also looked at the pages people clicked on when querying
for a medical term, to see if the authors of these pages provided
alternative descriptions of medical terms. To do this, we checked
for sentences that mentioned a medical term (e.g., "diplopia")
together with a word that recurred in many other pages. This
helped us enrich the dictionary of laypersons' synonyms even
further. A close inspection of the dictionary we built using these
two methods, conducted by three medical professionals, confirmed that 88 percent of the synonyms were indeed likely
descriptions of the corresponding medical term.

Armed with our new dictionary of many of the wonderful
ways in which people describe their symptoms, we counted how
many people queried for each of the symptoms, then divided
these people in two ways. First, we partitioned them into those
who asked about the drug we were analyzing. Second, we asked
how many people inquired about a symptom after they had
inquired about the drug and how many did so before they had
inquired about the drug. For those who had not asked about the
drug, we selected the middle of the period for which we collected the data, and counted the number of inquiries about the
adverse reaction before and after that date. We scored each
symptom for the likelihood that its appearance after queries for
the drug saw a significant increase by comparing it against the
number of queries for it before the query for the drug. We also
compensated for seasonal effects by comparing the increase
against the increase in the population that had not mentioned
the drug.

This procedure gives a score for each drug and each symptom.
To make sure that the scores we give are not spurious, random

numbers, we compared those scores against data collected by other means. One source of data for such comparisons is the FAERS reports. It turns out that for most of the best-selling drugs in the United States the correlation between the score we compute using data from search engines and the number of reports of symptoms and drugs in FAERS is reasonably high and is not likely to be a random fluke. However, there is a snag: Some of the symptoms that appear frequently in FAERS are rarely queried for in search engines, and vice versa—that is, some symptoms that receive high scores in search-engine data are almost never reported to FAERS, and some symptoms for which there are plenty of reports on FAERS received a low score in our search-engine data. When we tried to understand that discrepancy, we noticed a few things. First, no matter what drugs we looked at, the symptoms that were outliers either in FAERS or in search-engine data always appeared as outliers in one of them, but never in the other. Second, the outlier symptoms in FAERS were more serious symptoms, such as diarrhea, nausea, chest pain, and dizziness. The outlier symptoms in search-engine data were more benign—for example, sleepiness, weight gain, and general weakness. Finally, we noticed that, on average, people tended to query about the search-engine outliers at a much later time after querying for the drug, relative to the FAERS outliers.

All these findings lead us to believe that the outliers represent two distinct ways in which side effects are experienced. First, someone who experiences chest pain or diarrhea shortly after beginning to take a drug is likely to associate the side effect with the drug and to report the side effect to his or her doctor and perhaps to the FDA. This is especially true if the side effect is severe and if the person goes to an emergency room. However, when a side effect appears a long time after someone begins taking a drug, and if that side effect is not severe, one may not even make the association between the drug and the side effect, even if he decides to complain to his doctor. Instead, he may think of it as a new condition.

What we have discovered, then, is not just a new way of eliciting information on side effects, but a new class of side effects that have so far eluded discovery because of their longer appearance time and their milder appearance. Such side effects are not likely to surface even when websites such as the ones I described above are used, because they still rely on people to associate a drug and a side effect—a drawback that the use of search-engine data overcomes through the long-term association of people's searches.

Another class of medicines that the same procedures can be applied to, and that might benefit even more from additional evidence to their safety, is vaccines. Vaccination is one of the most successful public-health campaigns in recorded history. According to some estimates, it has prevented more than 100 million cases of contagious disease in the United States alone.[9] Almost from the start of vaccination campaigns, and growing in proportion to their size, a vocal anti-vaccination movement has sprung up. Often this movement plays into the fears of parents, amplifying rare adverse events and glossing over the benefits of vaccines. After all, there is something strange about taking a perfectly healthy baby to a nurse for shots that can cause fever and perhaps more serious conditions. Most new parents today probably have never met a person crippled by polio, or known of someone who has died from measles. We have forgotten the iron lungs and sanitariums. And in any case, with vaccination it pays to be a free rider. If everyone else got vaccinated, you probably could safely forgo it, because the chance of an epidemic would be small.

It is therefore not surprising that purveyors of anti-vaccination information have been successful in their attempts. A case in point is the debunked 1998 study by Dr. Andrew Wakefield and his colleagues which suggested that there might be a link between the Measles-Mumps-Rubella (MMR) vaccine and autism. Though that study has been retracted from the journal *Lancet*, which originally published it, its effects are still very much felt. Search the Internet and you will find plenty of sites which will tell you why that study is still valid. And in the physical world, MMR vaccination rates, which had reached 92 percent in the United Kingdom, had by 2002 fallen to 65 percent in some areas.[10] The effect of this decrease were immediate. Outbreaks of measles, unheard of for more than a decade, had returned to the UK, and there had been several deaths.

After developing our system for finding side effects of medical drugs, we also applied it to vaccinations. What we found were mostly symptoms that any parent would be aware of. The short-term symptoms, which were more likely reported to the FDA, were fever, diarrhea, and nausea. The long-term ones, more prominent in search-engine data, were weight loss and tiredness. Thus, our modest contribution to the controversy over vaccination is that our data do not support the claim that vaccines represent a long-term risk. This is in line with many other studies, using a variety of data and research methodologies, that have not shown vaccines to represent a significant hazard.

In discovering the side effects of drugs, the first date of importance is when the person first received the drug. Our main interest is to look for unusual and unexpected medical phenomena after that date. However, perhaps we can also go back in time and try to determine what got a person to take the drug in the first place—that is, what are some of the precursors of his or her medical condition.

When we recognize that someone has a medical condition, we can go back in time and see what unusual occurrence happened to that person recently. Some of these things will be related to happenings associate with the condition—for example, the reason an ambulance ride usually occurs shortly before someone is diagnosed as suffering from a heart attack is not that ambulances cause heart attacks, but that ambulances are used to ferry people with suspected heart attacks to a hospital. The more interesting things that happen before a person is diagnosed with a disease are the risk factors—that is, things that happen before the disease and that are part of the process that cause it. An example of the latter is smoking, which causes lung cancer. Distinguishing between a risk factor and an event associated with the disease requires elaborate experimentation. I wanted to focus on finding candidates for further scrutiny by epidemiologists.

Looking into the past to find risk factors for disease

Modern epidemiology probably started with John Snow. In 1854, London experienced a serious outbreak of cholera, which was eventually to kill about 600 people. At the time, the prevailing theory was that cholera was caused by "bad air." Snow was suspicious of that theory. After talking to people in the areas of London most affected by cholera, Snow concluded that transmission of cholera happened through water, specifically a pump on Broad Street. "It will be observed," wrote Snow, "that the deaths either very much diminished, or ceased altogether, at every point where it becomes decidedly nearer to send to another pump than to the one in Broad Street."[11] Though he could not detect anything wrong using chemical tests or his microscope, he convinced the local council to remove the handle of the pump in Broad Street, thereby stopping the disease by preventing new infections. Later he also plotted the cases of cholera on a map, thereby providing even more compelling evidence that water from the Broad Street pump was to blame.

Today, risk factors for various diseases and conditions are found in both the physical world and the virtual one. For example, will joining an online dating site increase one's risk of contracting a sexually transmitted disease? Does being active on Facebook put one at a higher risk for depression? Obviously, we could use Snow's methods, interview a few hundred people, and test whether this is true or not. But then for every new risk factor that we thought was out there we would have to find a few hundred people, interview them, and then analyze the data. Instead, we could scan a large population for every conceivable risk factor and then test all the possible combinations at once. By now it should be obvious that we should be able to do this using search data. Unfortunately, that entails three problems. First, how would we find a group of search-engine users who are suffering from the medical condition we are interested in researching? Second, how could we interpret their search queries in a wider sense? When a user asks about "Woodstock," we would like to test not only if participating in a specific rock festival that took place near the Catskill region of New York State in 1969 is a risk factor for the condition we are interested in, but also if rock concerts in general are a risk factor, or perhaps if being in that part of New York is a risk factor. What we really want is some way to interpret search-engine queries in their wider sense. Third, how would we test whether the risk factors referred to in the queries lead to a higher risk for the condition?

The first problem—that of finding a group of search-engine users who are suffering from the medical condition we are interested in researching—troubled us for a long time. The problem is that we cannot directly ask users of a search engine if they are suffering from a certain medical condition. This would be a major breach of privacy, and we would not be likely to get a response anyway. After pondering lots of ideas, we finally realized that some users' search queries would be helpful. Although the average search query is only three words long, some queries are very detailed. Indeed, some users begin their queries by telling the search engine what is troubling them. For example, users might ask: "I am pregnant. Can I drink one glass of wine?" Such queries, though rare, directly identify a small set of users who have specific conditions. This is what I will refer to as a *high-precision* group of people—that is, a group in which it is highly likely that all the members have the medical condition we are interested in. Granted, it does not include all the people who have that condition. Some people with the condition, perhaps most of them, do not identify as having a condition and will not be put into the high-precision group. But the high-precision group is a good starting point for building an automatic method that will scan queries submitted by other people and decide whether they have the medical condition of interest.

Before we can do that, we need to ask what kind of search-engine queries would give us the most information about a person's condition. We limit ourselves to queries of a medical nature (that is, questions about symptoms, diseases, and medical drugs), and give this list of queries to a learning algorithm—a computer program that, in this case, takes a list of all the medical queries that a person made to a search engine and the condition the person identified himself or herself as having, and tries to find some rule that will be able to say confidently what disease the person has.

Let me take a short detour to explain a little about learning algorithms—that is, computer programs that learn. Learning algorithms are a thing of wonder. In recent years their popularity has increased with the quantities of digital data that are generated. Today they can warn a driver that a pedestrian is jumping into the road, read checks, guide autonomous cars, and recommend movies and books at Amazon.

The origin of learning algorithms is often attributed to a paper published in 1950 by Alan Turing, a British mathematician. In that paper, titled "Computing machinery and intelligence,"[12] Turing addressed the question whether machines can think—a seemingly simple question until you begin to try to define what a machine is and what thinking is. Instead of trying to define these concepts, Turing changed the question. He asked whether a machine could win what he called the Imitation Game. In the Imitation Game, the machine is enclosed in one room, a human player of the game in another, and a human judge in a third. The judge can ask both the machine and the human player questions by typing them into a terminal, and the two players can respond through the terminal. The goal of the judge is to decide which room houses the computer, and the machine does its best to fool the judge. If the machine is able to do this, it has won the game. Essentially, Turing replaced the original question ("Can machines think?") with the question "Can machines act indistinguishably from humans?" His game has become known as the Turing Test.

For some time after the Turing Test was devised, some people thought that computers soon would be able to "pass" it. In 1965, Herbert Simon offered this prediction: "machines will be capable, within twenty years, of doing any work a man can do."[13] For better or worse, things have not turned out that way, and computers have yet to beat humans in a Turing Test. Therefore, a more modest approach has been taken in recent years in the field of Machine Learning. Here, the goal is not to beat humans in a Turing Test. Instead, it is to build computer programs that can learn from experience without being specifically programmed to do it. Experience, in this case, may be the results of its interaction with the world, as it is run, or data that was collected in the past. For example, a Machine Learning algorithm might observe which email messages you mark as spam, and decide how to classify future messages as spam or not spam. Another algorithm might learn how you divide your email messages into folders and do that automatically for you the next time a message comes in.

Machine Learning algorithms aim to generalize from the examples they are shown. For example, such an algorithm will not learn that a specific message is spam, but it may learn that if a message contains the words "transfer money" it is likely to be spam. Whereas humans are good at making generalizations from a small number of samples, Machine Learning algorithms are good at making them from huge amounts of data. It is estimated that between 88 percent and 90 percent of the email messages sent are spam.[14] Reading even a small sample of them and writing rules to decide which are spam and which are not would be prohibitively expensive and time consuming, but Machine Learning algorithms do so effectively, adapting to new kinds of spam and saving us from a deluge of it.

But how do these algorithms learn? Some intuition can be gotten from the most basic Machine Learning algorithm, called the Perceptron. Let's return to the example of classifying email messages according to whether or not they contain spam. To train our algorithm, we begin with a set of the email messages that have been annotated by a human expert, who has marked each one of them as either spam or not spam. Next, we need to represent each message as a set of numbers, because computers find it difficult to interpret texts. One way this is commonly done is by counting the number of times each word occurs in a message. Each word described in this way is called an *attribute*. Because the English language contains many distinct words, it may be necessary to use hundreds of thousands or even millions of distinct words to represent the complete set of messages. However, each message only contains a small subset of the possible words. The task of our algorithm to find some combination of these counts of words such that if they exceed a certain threshold we will say that the message in question is spam and if it does not exceed that certain threshold we will say that the message is legitimate. An easy way to combine the count of words is by giving each word a weight and adding up the multiplication of weights by counts. The algorithm simply needs to find what the best weights are. It does so by first assigning some random weight to each word, then adjusting the weights by examining the messages one by one. For example, it takes the first message, computes the score of that message (by multiplying the weights by the counts of words), and predicts whether that message is spam by whether its score exceeds the threshold. It then goes back and compares its prediction against the human expert's decision. If the prediction was correct, no adjustment of the weights is necessary. If the prediction was incorrect, the weights are adjusted so the next time a similar message would be shown to the algorithm, it would make a correct decision. This process is then repeated by showing the algorithm millions of email messages until it no longer makes too many mistakes.

Let us now return to our original question of how to examine queries in which users of search engines mention medical terms, and decide what diseases or conditions the users are suffering from.[15] To make the problem simpler, we will not assume that a person can have *any* disease. Instead, our algorithm will try to predict if the condition a person asks about most frequently is the condition that the person has. Someone who is suffering from HIV might also ask about AIDS or even about the flu, so simply deciding according to what conditions is asked about most frequently may not work. But by providing the algorithm with a count of how many times a person asked about each medical condition, we give the algorithm much more information to work with, hoping that it will provide a better decision. Just as in the earlier example we had an expert who labeled email messages as spam, here we can use the people who identified themselves as suffering from certain conditions as the experts. To measure the accuracy of our algorithms, we can look at how many of those self-identified users our algorithm labeled correctly. But we can also use the information collected by the Centers for Disease Control on the number of cases that were identified in the United States for certain diseases which the CDC deems important enough to track. These include various cancers and infectious diseases. When we did so, we found that our algorithm could indeed pinpoint a high-accuracy group of users for a large number of diseases.

Some algorithms allow us to look into their decision-making processes. For example, we can see which words get the highest score for making a decision. Our algorithm looked at both the medical condition asked about most frequently and the one asked about with the second highest frequency, and found that a high ratio between the two was a strong indicator of a person's condition.

Having solved the first part of the problem, we can now proceed to the second: interpreting queries in their wider sense. As I mentioned before, we assume that there is some likelihood that a person who queries a certain location or activity is at the location or participates in the activity. But we want to interpret an activity by its various facets. Moving to a new house means not only a new premises. It can also mean a new location, new furniture, a new school, and a new job. Somehow we want to represent the fact that a person asks about a new house in a way that the computer algorithm will be able to test each of those aspects. If I develop a new allergy, is it because of something in the house, or because of the new furniture I bought?

Once again we turn to search-engine users for help. People who contribute to Wikipedia write the entries in that online encyclopedia and annotate each entry with a set of categories. We can make use of these categories by mapping queries to Wikipedia entries, much as we built our dictionary of synonyms for medical symptoms earlier in this chapter. This means that when a person queries for "Burning Man" we will assume that there is some chance that he or she will end up going to that festival and thus will take part in an event in Black Rock Desert, an event in Nevada, a clothing-optional event, a public nudity event, and a counterculture festival, to name but a few of the categories used in Wikipedia to describe Burning Man. If

Burning Man represents a risk factor for some medical condition, it could be that other events in Nevada pose a similar risk.
By relating the events to a wider sense of attributes we allow our
algorithms to capture this commonality.

At this stage we have found are set of users who are very likely
suffering from the medical condition in which we are interested,
and have represented their queries with a large set of descriptions. Now we want to use these data to search for common
attributes among these people. We would like to find what happened shortly before a person identified as having a condition,
or querying about it. These are the precursors we are looking
for. In epidemiology there are two major approaches to doing
this. The first is to compare all the people who are suffering from
a condition against similar people who are not suffering from
the condition. If I take a group of people who are suffering from
lung cancer and compare them against a group of people of similar age, income, race, education, and so forth, I may be able to
show that the first group differs from the second in that many
more of them smoke cigarettes. What is tricky about such an
analysis is finding similar people. This is especially true of the
Internet, where any information we have on demographics is
only an estimate. Instead, we opted for the approach in which
each person is compared against himself or herself at other
times. That approach is useful if we can observe people for a relatively long period of time and compare the time long before they
develop their condition against the period just before that
period. Intuitively, if there was a major change in their behavior
or their lifestyle just before the condition developed, it may be
that this change is to blame for a condition. This approach is the
one that is commonly used to decide whether vaccinations are
safe for use.

What do the data show? We have looked at several medical conditions, and the results seem to indicate that we can indeed identify interesting precursors—specifically ones that appear a short time before a disease occurs.

Many of the precursors our system identified are not risk factors for disease (that is, things people do that put them in harm's way for a disease or cause it to erupt). Instead, they are things that happen before the medical condition appears or before a person admits to having the condition. For example, before an abortion people search for Planned Parenthood, an organization that, among other services, provides abortions. It is not that Planned Parenthood causes abortions, but that women who decide to have an abortion check out Planned Parenthood. Similarly, women identified as pregnant by the algorithm searched for the symptoms of pregnancy.

In other cases our data showed some interesting hints about possible risk factors—that is, things that people search for that can indeed be a cause of a disease. We found that before developing an allergy, people search for pet stores and certain cereals. Both pets and cereals are suspected of being allergens and appear in the medical literature that deals with allergies. Users we identified as having an eating disorder search for, among others, images and depression. Recall our discussion of anorexia in the preceding chapter and you will not be surprised.

All these examples may have been detectable through analysis of activity in the physical world. The next two conditions showed precursors that have not been identified there. Herpes, a sexually transmitted infection, has become more prevalent in recent years. In our data we found that users who we identified as suffering from herpes tended to search for heterosexual online dating sites and pornography. Perhaps similarly, those people who our algorithms identified as suffering from HIV search for online pornography and homosexual dating sites. It is not far-fetched to believe that people who meet new partners in online dating are more at risk for developing a sexually transmitted infection, but until now there has been scant evidence that such is the case. We are not sure how pornography contributes as a risk factor—perhaps it is only a precursor. Validating our results and deciding whether the phenomena in question are precursors or risk factors will require further experiments by experts.

Now that we have developed a method that requires very little human effort, it could easily continue to work day in and day out scanning a whole gamut of medical conditions. The only limitation is that enough people with a condition will have to contribute queries. But the benefit of such a system could be enormous. New risk factors could be discovered almost immediately, and health authorities could be informed. Imagine how useful such a system could be if it could quickly discover that people who searched for a specific type of food or a specific place suddenly developed a specific infectious disease, such as the flu.

So far this chapter has described two kinds of research that bear on peoples' medical conditions. In the case of drug side effects, the algorithms look at the time from which a person takes a drug and into the future. With risk factors, we looked back from the time a person was diagnosed with a disease, and tried to find out what change may have caused the disease. In both cases, the time scale at which we were looking was months. Such long time scales are one advantage of Internet data. Sometimes, however, what is needed is an algorithm that can rapidly detect an outbreak of a disease and tell health authorities about it.

What happens in Vegas doesn't always stay in Vegas

In many cases information about a new outbreak of some infectious disease can be found, but only in retrospect. The problem is that on any given day there are many signs that could be interpreted as an outbreak of the disease. But is the fact that ten people asked about the symptoms of the flu in in a city the size of New York a sign of an outbreak? Probably not. And even if it is, we may be able to wait a few more days before deciding to ring the alarm bells. Other diseases require a more vigilant eye, either because they are more virulent or because they are more dangerous.

Even before the Internet could be used to monitor disease outbreaks, people tried to use somewhat similar information to decide if an outbreak had begun. Weng-Keen Wong and colleagues did so by monitoring the hospitalization reports of hospital emergency rooms. In a paper titled "WSARE: What's strange about recent events?"[16] they described a statistical method for comparing these hospitalization reports over time and deciding when to raise alarm. The problem is that by the time hospitals report unusual lists of cases, it may be already too late.

A case in point is an outbreak of Severe Acute Respiratory Syndrome. SARS had been brewing in South China for several months when, in March 2003, a medical doctor traveled from mainland China to Hong Kong. He stayed at the Metropole Hotel in Kowloon, and, while there, infected 16 other guests at that hotel. Many of those guests then traveled abroad, and health authorities saw cases of SARS in Canada, Singapore, Taiwan, and Vietnam. By the time the outbreak was brought under control, 44 people had died in Canada, 33 in Singapore, 37 in Taiwan, and 5 in Vietnam.

During the first few days after the discovery of SARS in the four countries mentioned above, medical authorities were struggling to understand whether the infections had something in common and whether the disease had already spread to many other countries beyond those four. Epidemiologists had to interrogate each of the patients and try to work back in time to see if they had ever met one of the others or been in the same place as one of them. Their investigations led back to the Metropole. Thinking about this problem, we wanted to know whether we could use Internet data to provide a rapid-alert system that would also take into account of people's movements around the world, or even just their movements within their own countries.

To test our ideas[17] we decided to examine events at which large numbers of people come into close contact, such as rock festivals and religious festivals. Some such festivals are truly gigantic. The Kumbh Mela, a Hindu festival that takes place once every three years, drew more than 100 million people in 2013.[18] In 2012 the yearly Muslim Hajj was attended by more than 3 million. When so many people come together in close quarters under conditions that are not optimal in terms of sanitation, lodging, and food, it doesn't take much more than a single individual who came to the festival carrying an infectious disease to cause the infection of many others.

Our idea was to try to do two things simultaneously: (1) identify a group of people who were likely to attend a mass gathering and (2) determine whether members of that group described suffering from a disease that was unusual because the individuals in question had not had the symptoms of it before going to the festival or because only people who had attended the festival discussed the symptoms of the disease.

Just as we did with the side effects of drugs, we searched for all the ways in which people described symptoms. This time we used two sources of data. We assumed that people are likely to tell the world when they attend a festival. For this reason we looked at data from Twitter. Unfortunately, as you may recall from the earlier chapters, most people are squeamish about discussing their medical problems in an identifiable forum such as Twitter. So to supplement this source of information, we again turned to search engines' query logs, where medical symptoms were more likely to appear but where the fact that a person attended a festival might not. Our hope was that by simultaneously tracking data from both sources we would overcome the weakness of each separate source.

We used data on ten events that occurred in the second half of 2012: the Hajj and nine music festivals held in Britain. On average, about 14,000 people attended each of these festivals and mentioned this fact on Twitter. Our search-engine logs were somewhat sparser, because we could only identify approximately 5,600 users who were very likely to have been at each of the festivals. As was noted above, people are more likely to tweet that they attended a festival than to use a search engine to ask about it in a way that allows us to be sure that they attended the festival.

Our analysis, which compared the symptoms users mentioned before the festival against those mentioned after the festival and also compared the symptoms that users mentioned against the symptoms that other people in close geographical proximity mentioned, turned up some rather interesting information. For example, a mild but very common symptom that attendees described after most festivals was being tired. Anyone who has been to a rock festival should not be surprised by this finding, especially as it turned up in the analysis of the Twitter data. More surprising, perhaps, is that several people complained of coughs after a certain festival. Those complaints may have been due to respiratory illness contracted during the festival. After another festival, many people complained about depression. We can only speculate whether that was because the festival had been good or because of chemicals the participants had consumed.

All the examples above turned up in our analysis of Twitter data, and are mostly of symptoms which people feel they can describe on Twitter. In the search-engine data, somewhat more sensitive symptoms were mentioned. Vomiting and diarrhea were queried by people who had just returned from the several of the festivals, as were fever and headaches. Apparently these two data sources—search-engine queries and tweets—are complementary in the diseases that can be expected to be mentioned on them. Both, however, turned out to be a valuable data source for pinpointing not only the appearance of a disease but also its source, in this case a festival. Moreover, the continuous analysis of this data could quickly raise an alarm with health authorities.

The vast amount of Internet data provides an unprecedented opportunity to improve public health by monitoring the adverse effects of medicines, new risk factors for diseases, and outbreaks of infectious diseases. Though Internet data are less accurate than data collected at medical facilities, their volume and their immediacy make them useful. The fact that people often go online to search for information before they visit a doctor makes rapid discovery of their medical problems practicable.

5 What Patients Want to Know About Their Disease, and How Information from the Internet Can Help Them

In 1995, Jean-Dominique Bauby, the 43-year-old editor in chief of the fashion magazine Elle, *suffered a stroke. His mental capacity undiminished, he was paralyzed in all but a few of his facial muscles. With the help of an assistant he wrote a memoir titled* The Diving Bell and the Butterfly.[1] *In it he describes his condition a few months after his stroke: "I am fading away. Slowly but surely. Like the sailor who watches the home shore gradually disappear, I watch my past recede. My old life still burns within me, but more and more of it is reduced to the ashes of memory."*

When you live with a disease for a long time, it can sometimes be easy to forget what life looked like before the disease struck. Trying to learn about a disease, its treatment options, and other information can be a full-time job, not only for the person who has been taken ill but often also for that person's friends and family members. To some extent, people need to build a new role in their lives. This role, unwanted and uninvited, grows and shrinks over time. It has many aspects to it: some shared with the treating doctor, some not. In this chapter I will describe work in which we tried to characterize how people deal with their condition, and to use it as a means of helping doctors to treat patients and helping patients to better understand their predicament.

Quantifying the five stages of grief

In her 1973 book *Coping with Death and Dying,*[2] Elisabeth Kübler-Ross described what happens when someone receives a piece of really bad news—for example, news that that he or she has a serious disease or has failed an important test at school, or that a loved one has died. Kübler-Ross suggested that people pass through five stages as they try to come to grips with the new reality. Her description, which became known as the "five stages of grief" model, had people start with denial of the news, then express anger, followed by bargaining, depression, and acceptance. In the denial stage, a patient may say something like "That's impossible; you must have the wrong diagnosis." Then, after expressing anger at being so diagnosed, the patient may try to bargain with reality. A religious person may try to barter recovery for more observance. ("If God helps me recover, I will be more observant.") The next step in coming to grips with a terrible reality is depression, followed, finally, by acceptance of the condition.

Many medical practitioners who are asked about the Kübler-Ross model agree that, broadly, it is correct. That is, people might skip some stages, and may go back and forth between stages. Generally, however, the model is taken to be correct. But how do they know this, beyond their personal, anecdotal, experience? A search of the scientific literature reveals that about 8,000 scientific papers mention this model, some substantiating it through qualitative data. By this point in the present book, you will have realized that I prefer a more quantitative approach to life. Here, sadly, the literature is lacking.

What would one have to do to validate the Kübler-Ross model in a quantitative manner? A simple way would be to have an experimenter (perhaps a graduate student) sit outside the office of an oncologist and wait for people who emerge from the office, having been told that they have been diagnosed with cancer. The student would ask each patient—whose life had just been turned upside down—to answer a set of questions about his (or her) state of mind, and then to complete the same survey once every few hours so that his state of mind could be tracked as he passed through the stages.

Even less challenging psychological studies find it difficult to recruit participants. In one study,[3] researchers tried to get the parents of children newly diagnosed with cancer to participate in six sessions designed to assist them in coping with the child's disease. As the researchers reported, many parents were unwilling or unable to do this because they were "feeling overwhelmed." They had bigger problems on their minds than helping to validate a psychological model, even if it was for their own benefit.

Yishai Ofran, Dan Pelleg, and I thought we had a better idea.[4] We would identify people who had just been diagnosed with cancer and who were searching the Internet for information about it. By classifying the pages they read or the queries they made as they searched for information and were indicative of one or another of the stages of grief, we would see whether they indeed passed through the five stages.

Identifying people who had been diagnosed with cancer, or whose family members or friends had been so diagnosed, was simple. We looked for people who suddenly developed an intense interest in a specific type of cancer. For example, people who, suddenly, began searching for information about colon cancer, and kept doing so for a number of days. Having found such a group, we discovered that about 6,000 Web pages were read by many of the people in it. Our next step was to ask a few psychologists "What would a person in the denial stage (or the depression stage) read?" This, it turns out, is a difficult question— so difficult that we could not get a consensus among the psychologists on how to identify the stage people were in according to the pages they were reading.

We had to reconsider the plan of our study. The problem, essentially, was that it was impossible to decide which pages were read when people were in the different stages (assuming that, indeed, these stages exist). But perhaps we could divide these pages into more easily identifiable categories, for example according to whether they dealt with treatments of cancer, with support networks, or with diagnosis.

Because the sheer volume of the data would require several weeks of work by a single person, we turned to a tool that is often used by Internet companies, though rarely discussed. Even though many of the tasks that operators of search engines and online merchants must perform are completely automated others are extremely difficult for a computer, though they are rather easy for a human to perform. For example, finding the price of an item shown in the Web page of an online store is quite hard for a computer but very easy for a human. This is where Amazon's Mechanical Turk (and other similar services) come into play. Mechanical Turk is a market in which the product traded is human effort. Its name comes from a chess-playing machine, constructed in 1770, that purportedly could play at a high level against a human opponent but was later revealed to house a human who moved the pieces.

Companies use Mechanical Turk, for example, to have the text extracted from a large number of pictures showing street signs, agreeing to pay a cent or a dime for each image that a person processes. A task may take a few seconds, so the pay is appropriate, and people all over the world, but predominantly from the United States and India, will perform such tasks. Because even a human makes mistakes, the same task is usually sent to several people, after which the most common answer given by them is used. This is a cheap and effective way to solve tasks that require intensive human effort.[5]

Using Mechanical Turk, we divided our 6,000 pages into eleven general categories within a few days. These were categories that were easy for a layperson to decide on, including a description of symptoms, being the page of a support group, or a list of treatments for cancer. We then had to decide how to link our eleven categories to any of Kübler-Ross's five stages. It turns out that there is a mathematical tool that can do exactly that.

Starting with work done by the Russian mathematician Andrei Markov late in the nineteenth century, extensive study has been devoted to understanding systems that move through different states, or conditions. The model inspired by Markov's work, known as a Markov Model, describes a system whose next state depends only on its current state. For example, such a system could be the weather in my area, and the states could be "rainy," "dry," and "snowy." If today is dry, a Markov Model can specify the probability that tomorrow will be rainy, snowy, or dry. However, tomorrow's weather does not explicitly depend on yesterday's.

A later improvement on the basic Markov Model came in the late 1960s with the work of Leonard Baum and his colleagues at the Institute for Defense Analyses in Princeton. Instead of assuming that they knew what state a system was in, Baum and colleagues tried to look at a system whose states were invisible, so that the only information one could observe was some indication of the system's state. In the case of the weather example mentioned in the preceding paragraph, a Hidden Markov Model (as Baum's system came to be known) would occur when I could not look outside to see the weather. Instead, I could watch to see if the clothes worn by people who come to the house were wet, and assume that if they were wet there was some probability that it was raining outside, but there was some other probability they had been drenched by sprinklers that had gone into action after a long spell of dry weather. More generally, when a system is in a specific hidden state, it generates corresponding visible outputs.

Though Hidden Markov Models may seem very abstract, they have found many uses in many areas, including speech recognition, bioinformatics, and cryptanalysis. In our case, they provide a solution to our mapping problem. Let us assume that people pass through some distinct mental stages during their grief, and that in each stage they encounter different information needs. These needs are apparent from the pages they read. In analogy to the Hidden Markov Model, the hidden states correspond to the mental stages between which people transition; the visible states are the subjects of the pages that people read, as classified by the Mechanical Turk workers. All the visible states may appear when people are in different hidden states, but the probability that each state will appear is different.

One drawback of using Hidden Markov Models is that it is difficult to associate a specific hidden state with one of Kübler-Ross's five stages. But if the data support the use of a model with distinct transitions, such an association may not be overly important.

Using search-engine queries submitted to the Yahoo engine during a six months period by 20,808 people, we tried to fit the best Hidden Markov Model to the pages people read as results of their queries. Fitting a model means guessing the number of hidden states in a model and then, using a different subset of the data, finding the probabilities that people will move from one state to the other and the probabilities that they will read a page of a given topic when in that state. The quality of the model is assessed by testing how well the model describes the observed behaviors in the remainder of the data.

The best model turns out to be one that has exactly five hidden stages. This, though indirect, is one of the first quantitative pieces of evidence for a 40-year-old model. More interesting are the details of this model. Once we saw that a Hidden Markov Model is indeed a good way to describe the search behaviors we had observed, we built separate models for people who asked about acute forms of cancer and for people who asked about more chronic cancers, the two groups being defined according to rates of survival.

The two models turn out to be very different. The model that describes the behavior of people searching for information on acute cancers tends to see people remaining in the first three stages, and the behavior of such people is more string-like than that of people searching for information on chronic cancers (that is, they are less likely to go back to earlier stages). People asking about chronic cancers much prefer the latter two stages, and tend to stay in them longer than those suffering from acute cancers. The stages also differ in the information people seek: in cases of chronic cancers social support is an important topic, whereas in cases of acute cancers treatment options feature prominently.

We had one more interesting phenomenon to investigate, though it did not bear on the five stages of grief. Yahoo runs one of the most extensive social networks on the Internet, a network that allows people to chat via text or voice. We overlaid this network on the search data and examined how the searches of friends of people diagnosed with cancer looked when they searched for information about cancer.

A first sign that something interesting happens between friends is our observation that if two friends on Yahoo's network searched for information on a specific type of cancer, they were more than twice as likely to search for information on the same type of cancer as would be expected to occur by chance. We again divided the population into two groups according to the severity of the cancer they were seeking information about. In cases of aggressive cancer, both people in a pair searched for about twelve days, and the second person began to search nine days after the first person began to do so. In cases of less aggressive cancers, the first person to begin searching also searched for about twelve days; the friend began searching fifteen days later and searched for only five days.

The first of a pair of friends to begin searching was also more likely than the second to be interested in treatments for cancer and in general information about the disease. The second person to begin searching was more likely to look for pages related to the causes of cancer and for pages promising help with social support.

We believe that the first of a pair of friends to begin searching is either the patient or a close family member. Such people begin searching once they know they have cancer, or are informed of a strong suspicion to that effect. Friends and more distant relatives begin searching later. People who have been diagnosed with acute cancers have less time to search for information because they need to begin treatment; their friends do the searching for them, as is evident from the longer search periods of the second searchers. In cases of less acute cancers, the patient can afford to search for information for a longer time, and after a relatively short search a friends may decide that the disease is not as severe as had been thought.

Why are these findings interesting, beyond giving some support to the five-stages-of-grief model? I believe that the data provide an important and otherwise difficult to obtain insight into the critical period that follows diagnosis. During that short period (which our data suggest is well under two weeks), people are thirsty for information, but their information needs change rapidly as they transition between stages. Medical doctors and nurses should recognize this, and should provide information in a way that is aligned with patients' needs, emphasizing some aspects of the information more than others. Moreover, it is important to understand what stage a patient is in, perhaps by asking the patient some guiding questions or listening to his or her concerns (even non-medical concerns) just to detect what phase of his or her information seeking the patient is at, and to provide information appropriately.

According to our data, the kind of information someone needs during the first few days after that person or a close loved one has been diagnosed with cancer changes rapidly. It changes, most probably, for several reasons: First, the person's grappling with the new condition changes as the person goes though the five stages of grief. Second, as someone learns more about his or her disease, the person may want to gain an even deeper understanding of specific facets of the disease, or of particular treatment options. Therefore, after a doctor informs a patient of a cancer diagnosis, it may well be more beneficial for the doctor to schedule several short meetings over the following days to discuss the disease and the options for treatment than for the doctor to give the patient all the information the doctor considers necessary at once. Although we have not studied much longer periods of information seeking, it is likely that similar patterns appear during such periods. Treatment can take months or years. Over such time spans, what people want to learn, and in how much detail, is likely to change. Doctors, who are the primary source of authoritative information and are often aware of patients' thirst for information, should be attentive to such changes in interest.

Information providers on the Internet should also tailor their information according to patients' needs and interests. For example, the pages devoted to specific cancers on many medical websites[6] begin with symptoms, causes, and risk factors. However, a person who already has been diagnosed with a cancer will have very little use for these materials. He already knows that he has the disease. Websites should cater to people already diagnosed with a disease in a way that takes their mental states into account. As we have learned from our data, people with different mental states require different information, and their mental state changes rapidly in the first few days after diagnosis.

Medical investigation based on Internet data has several advantages over more traditional medical investigation. First, it enables researchers to learn about people's needs in a way that does not disrupt their activities, especially at a time of great mental burden. Second, it gives patients empowering information. Some patients want to know everything about their condition; others prefer only the bare minimum. Distinguishing between these two categories of patients and knowing what information to give patients in each of them is difficult, and trial and error can cause anguish. This is where research that is based on the Internet data has an advantage over similar research done in the physical world. Another area of research for such advantages is that which deals with mental conditions.

Detecting mood swings from Internet queries

Mental diseases are unique in that they are defined not by the organ they affect, but by their symptoms. Whereas heart disease plainly afflicts the heart, we are only beginning to understand how depression affects the brain, or how the brain causes depression. As the psychologist Gary Greenberg said: "In medicine, if you go to a doctor and say 'I have a sore throat and a fever' he can't say 'You have a strep throat' at least until he takes a throat culture ... whereas if you go to a psychiatrist and you tell him your symptoms that's all they have to go on."[7]

Nevertheless, medicine defines some behaviors as mental illnesses. One of the best known of these is bipolar disorder (also known by its older name, manic depression). Bipolar disorder is characterized by a cycling of moods between a manic state and a depression. In a manic state, one feels aroused, full of energy and vitality. Unfortunately, soon enough a person with bipolar disorder makes a transition to depression, in which the person lacks interest in everyday life (or in life itself) and exhibits self-denigration. Kay Redfield Jamison, a psychologist who has suffered from bipolar disorder since childhood, described the disease as one that "distorts moods and thoughts, incites dreadful behaviors, destroys the basis of rational thought, and too often erodes the desire and will to live. It is an illness that is biological in its origins, yet one that feels psychological in the experience of it, an illness that is unique in conferring advantage and pleasure, yet one that brings in its wake almost unendurable suffering and, not infrequently, suicide."

To treat the mood swings that bipolar disorder causes, psychiatrists use a class of drugs known as *mood stabilizers*. The most common of these, and the oldest, is derived from the element lithium. The beneficial effects of lithium for patients with bipolar disorder were discovered in the late nineteenth century. They were then neglected and forgotten for about 80 years, until they were accidentally rediscovered in 1949 by the Australian psychiatrist John Cade. While the psychological effects of lithium lay forgotten, lithium salts were used for everything from a replacement for table salt to an ingredient in the beverage that later was named 7Up. (Lithium was banned as a food additive in 1948.)

Lithium's beneficial effect on stabilizing the mood swings experienced by people with bipolar disorder comes at a price. Lithium has quite a few side effects which affect some of the people taking it, including dry mouth, headaches, impairment of memory, hallucinations, and seizures.

In a memoir titled *Scattershot: My Bipolar Family*, David Lovelace (who has been a carpenter and a bookstore proprietor) wrote: "Compared to bipolar's magic, reality seems a raw deal. It's not just the boredom that makes recovery so difficult, it's the slow dawning pain that comes with sanity—the realization of illness, the humiliating scenes, the blown money and friendships and confidence. Depression seems almost inevitable. The pendulum swings back from transcendence in shards, a bloody, dangerous mess. Crazy high is better than crazy low. So we gamble, dump the pills, and stick it to the control freaks and doctors. They don't understand, we say. They just don't get it. They'll never be artists."[8]

Lithium usually must be taken daily. If it is effective, the patient does not experience manic or depressive episodes, but does feel the side effects. After a while a patient may reach a conclusion that she has overcome her illness and can therefore stop taking the pills, for all they do is cause the side effects. That may be a poor decision—once she has stopped taking lithium, she may again experience the symptoms of manic depression.

Eric Horvitz, Ryen White, and I began to ask whether we could we identify the mood swings associated with manic depressive episodes.[9] Indeed, if we could, would it be possible to predict that they will occur in certain patients in the near future, thereby encouraging patients to take their pills in time, or to warn their caregivers of impending mood-swing event?

Once again, we decided to collect the queries submitted by anonymous people (this time to the Bing search engine), focusing on those who asked about mood disorder or more specifically about the drugs used to treat mood disorder. We thought that people would ask about their drugs soon after they had been prescribed. However, after we had collected the data we noticed a strange phenomenon: Some users kept asking about their drugs repeatedly, once every few days, and especially about their side effects. For example, many users submitted the simple query "lithium's side effects." Could there be something special about these users, and about their numerous queries about their drugs, beyond our hypothesis that they would ask about their drugs soon after they had been prescribed?

Our first inkling that something unusual was afoot came when we looked at the topics people queried around the time that they asked about their drugs. Three topics seemed to be unusually popular either just before or just after queries about the drugs: nutrition, shopping, and pornography. For some reason, in the two or three days after asking about the drug for treating mood disorder, some people were looking for porn at more than twice their usual rate.

In an effort to understand the search behavior we were observing, we turned to a new way of using an old tool: a survey. With the help of a company that specializes in getting people to answer surveys on the Internet, mostly for marketing purposes, we recruited 272 people who reported taking drugs for mood disorder. We asked them about the drugs they were taking and about their disease, but what we were really interested in was the relationship between their disease and their online behavior. One question we asked was "Do you search online for information about your medication?" The vast majority answered "Yes," and slightly more than half said they had done so more than once in the past few months. The most common response to the question "When do you ask about your drugs?" was "When the drug was first prescribed." Other common answers were "When side effects are experienced" and "When I felt that the drug wasn't working."

Interestingly, about a quarter of the respondents said that they ask about their drugs when they felt that a manic or depressive episode was beginning. This suggests that, for a large number of the people who repeatedly ask about their drugs, such queries can hint at the onset of an episode. We also knew from the queries we saw that specific changes in behavior were happening around the time these queries were made, so we asked our survey respondents "What do you do online when you have a manic, and separately a depressive, episode?" We made sure to phrase this as an open question, so as not to lead respondents to the kinds of behavioral changes that we saw. When the answers came back, we were positively surprised. During depression, most people said, they refrained from browsing the Internet. In our data, such times should appear as periods of inactivity. In contrast, our survey respondents said that during manic episodes they looked for things that, they said, made them happy: online shopping (specifically of the unnecessary kind) and pornography. We interpret these answers as suggesting that a respondent who repeatedly asked about his or her drugs probably was experiencing a manic episode at the time. If that is correct, perhaps we can go back in time and see when the first signs of an episode occurred, and warn the patient of the impending crisis.

Because mood disorder events are characterized by deviations from normal behavior, either up toward mania or down into depression, we trained our Machine Learning classifier to look at deviations from the normal behavior of each individual. We classified each query that a respondent made into one of about sixty topics, then calculated the likelihood that each individual would ask about these topics on days that were neither those on which they mentioned a drug nor a few days preceding or immediately after those days. The wide range of topics included shopping, online gaming, tourism, and cooking. The likelihoods we computed served as a baseline for the things a person was usually interested in. We then looked at the topics about which our users queried on a given day and computed the difference between those topics and the normal profile of their topics.

In view of the deviations between likelihoods, we tried to see whether it would be possible to predict that a person would query about his or her drugs tomorrow, the day after, or the day after tomorrow. As we saw above, people ask about their drugs on days when they are very likely to be experiencing a manic or depressive episode. We expected that the farther into the future we would try to predict, the worse the performance of the Machine Learning classifier would be. In practice, the classifier found it nearly impossible to predict whether a user would ask about his or her drugs more than one day in the future.

But looking at the deviations between topics queried by a user on one day and whether that person would ask about his or her drugs the next day, we found that we could train a classifier to predict the latter from the former with quite reasonable accuracy. Even with our crude data, where we do not know if the person was actually experiencing a mood disorder event, but instead only have an indication of it, that is, our interpretation that days on which a user asks about their drugs are those days when they experience and events, we could still provide warning of an impending event.

Perhaps our findings are not very surprising. Munmun de Choudhury asked women to complete a questionnaire shortly after giving birth.[10] The survey was in fact a psychological evaluation used to detect postpartum depression. After the participants had completed the questionnaire, de Choudhury asked them to provide records of their Facebook activities before and shortly after they gave birth. By correlating the answers to the questionnaire with the Facebook activities, she demonstrated that postpartum depression could be predicted, though perhaps not yet with a high enough specificity.

Taken together, the studies discussed above provide insight into what could be an important application for cell phones and other mobile devices. Our hope is that in the not-so-distant future people who are at high risk for certain mental disorders will be able to download an application that will monitor their search queries and warn them or members of their families when the disease seems to be raising its head. These applications might start with a classifier trained on large populations, such as ours, and might then use feedback from each user to improve its future predictions. For example, an application that predicts when a manic or a depressive episode is likely might use our classifier that was trained for the "average user." If the application predicts that tomorrow there will be a manic episode and an episode fails to materialize, the user will be able to tell that to the classifier. Patients should also provide information on whether they took steps to mitigate an episode, as many patients do when they feel the onset of an episode. If a manic episode occurs and the application had not predicted it, this information will also benefit the classifier. Over time, the classifier will learn the behaviors of each person running the application and improve its predictions. Doctors and family members will also be able to provide input, the former by instructing the patient on what he or she should do when an episode is predicted (e.g., perhaps take another dose of medicine) and the latter by providing feedback on what were successful ways of dealing with manic or depressive episodes.

We are already seeing the beginnings of this revolution. Ginger.io, a startup company in San Francisco, uses smartphones to improve mental health care. According to that company's website, "Our app uses sensor data collected through the phone and self-reported information to identify people who may need help. Providers can use this data to deliver support to the right people at the right time—making care more timely, effective and engaging." Hundreds of companies are exploring how mobile phones and fitness trackers can collect useful data so as to learn about people's health and to improve it. Combining the lessons learned from such mobile devices with insights gained from much larger populations online should help to improve the accuracy of interventions in a way that either those lessons or those insights alone will not be able to accomplish.

Late in 2014 the Samaritans (a charity in the United Kingdom that provides emotional support and tries to help prevent suicide) launched a new cell-phone application called Samaritans Radar.[11] Once it has been installed on a phone, Samaritans Radar collects the usernames of people that the phone's owner follows on Twitter and monitors them for words and phrases that the Samaritans identify as related to depression—for example, "hate myself," "depressed," and "help me." When these words and phrases are identified, the Samaritans send the person who installed the app an email message suggesting ways to help a person who might be depressed.

Samaritans Radar was written with the best of intentions, but it is highly problematic in many ways. First, the accuracy of detecting a depressed person simply by looking for a few phrases is doubtful; for example, the wording of a message may be ironic or sarcastic. Second, and much more important, is the question of privacy. If a person did not agree to have his or her individual data acted upon, such intervention might lead to the opposite of the intended outcome, as happened with some of the well-intentioned anorexia interventions mentioned earlier in this book.

The future app described above requires specific consent on the sides of all those concerned. First, the patient must agree to have his or her data collected and acted upon. Second, the patient's caregiver or physician will have to agree to receive alert messages, because receiving such a message will, to a certain extent, require them to act. Moreover, the app does not provide the raw search data to caregivers. (A patient's doctor will not know about any seedy searches the patient may have conducted late at night.) Instead, it provides a signal based on aggregate information: According to his or her queries, the patient may be heading for a mood-disorder event.

Personalized medicine has been hailed as the next revolution in medical care.[12] Medicine, it is hoped, can be tailored to each of us by profiling our DNA and matching each of us to the treatment that is best for a person with such a DNA profile. In a way, the application proposed above could be a form of truly personalized medicine—one that will learn about an individual's behaviors and the best ways to deal with them, and will offer each individual a choice of treatments. Someday, perhaps, when lithium is prescribed to a patient, an application will also be prescribed to help the patient to experience a better outcome, see beyond his or her predicament, and lead a more normal life.

Epilogue

In 1948, the U.S. National Health Services began a ground-breaking experiment, recruiting more than 5,000 adults in the Massachusetts town of Framingham to share their medical histories with the researchers and to undergo physical and medical tests every two years. The Framingham Heart Study continues, with its third generation of participants. By analyzing data collected over more than 60 years, researchers have been able to demonstrate the dangers of smoking, high cholesterol, and elevated blood pressure, and answer a variety of other medical questions, detailed in more than 1,000 scientific papers.

The Framingham Heart Study is unique in duration and in scale. Tracking more than 5,000 people was difficult in the days before computers were widely used. Today the Framingham Heart Study is considered a high-quality study, though the sample is relatively small. In many countries the complete medical records of the entire population are already computerized, or will soon be, providing unprecedented insights for medical researchers. However, medical records only show snapshots of people's health at specific (and disparate) times. They are akin to short flashes of light in an otherwise dark night. In contrast, data from the Internet can be characterized as a pale light shining throughout the night.

The World Wide Web lends itself to large-scale data collection. This and the fact that our behavior online closely mirrors our behavior offline are two reasons for the main claim I make in this book: that Internet data change how medical research can and should be done. Perhaps in the future that claim will become even bolder, because we will have learned how to help people improve their health by observing their Internet behavior and providing appropriate information.

It is not that traditional medical research is obsolete. It is that behavioral data from the Web helps us to answer questions that are hard to answer otherwise. As we have seen, Internet data are of great use when the questions we want to answer are related to sensitive topics—to behaviors that happen predominantly on the Web and when truthfulness is hard to achieve in the real world.

Another reason why Internet data are highly useful for medical purposes is that they may come from hundreds of millions of people—in some cases, from a significant portion of patients with a certain condition or of those using a certain drug. Internet data can be analyzed continually and over long periods of time, and often allow segmentation by geographical location and demographics.

We are only beginning to understand the benefits of these data. At the same time, we struggle with the ethical and privacy implications of putting these data to use. Our understanding of how to take advantage of them is an evolving process that requires a vigilant public, a sensitive scientific community, and careful regulation. As our awareness of what is technically possible and what is ethically acceptable develops, so does recognition by the public of how our data reflect on ourselves in ways that would not have been possible a decade or two ago. This mutual understanding should, in my view, lead us to an open and evolving dialogue about the kinds of benefits that we would like to gain for sacrificing some of our privacy. At least in the domain of health, I believe, we have a lot to gain.

I anticipate that if we can achieve an appropriate balance between privacy and ethics, on the one hand, and usefulness, on the other, more and more Internet data will become available to the research community. This availability will make it easier to collect the data and will help health experts to gain insights from them. We are already seeing this trend in the form of aggregated search-engine queries made available by services such as Google Trends and Bing Search API—data that can be used by researchers to understand, for example, the risk of chronic disease.[1]

There are some parallels between the present state of research of Internet data and the state of research of the human genome a decade ago. In 2003, when the human genome was first sequenced, there were few publicly available genetic databases. Today, tools such as the GenBank sequence database provides access to an exponentially growing set of genetic sequences, available to anyone with Internet access. Advances in biology and computer science have vastly improved the tools used to process these sequences, making them readily available to a much wider community than was feasible only 10 years ago. My hope is that we will be able to advance the state of medical research that uses Internet data to where public databases will be available, providing a similar boon to researchers.

In "Pâté de foie gras," a short science fiction story published in 1956,[2] Isaac Asimov relates the tale of a scientist to whom a farmer gives a goose that lays golden eggs. The scientist and his colleagues try to understand how a goose can lay golden eggs. After conducting every conceivable test, he and his colleagues run out of ideas. They dare not kill the goose. At wits' end, the scientist suggests that they publish their problem as a science fiction story because "science fiction readers have ideas. ... And since we have no ideas of our own, since we're up a dead-end street, what can we lose?"

We are not up a dead-end street, nor are we out of ideas. In parallel to our efforts to enable a larger community to conduct medical research that makes use of Internet data, we are striving to better understand what can be done with Internet data and to advance the science needed to make use of them. Therefore, if this book has raised questions that you think Internet data can answer, why not go ahead and try to answer them, or contact me or any of the many other researchers quoted in this book? Perhaps we could work on it together.

Appendix: How Can One Gain Access to Internet Data?

If the ideas in this book have whet your appetite to collate some Internet data and do some medical research of your own, this appendix describes some of the ways you could try to collect some data. The nature of the Internet means that this appendix is likely to become obsolete sooner than any of the chapters. Nevertheless, I hope that it will be of use for at least several years after publication.

It is important to note that data obtained through channels other than the official ones, such as by "scraping" a website, may be illegal, depending on each website's terms of use. You are strongly advised to verify the legality of your actions (and their acceptance by a website's owner) before collecting data.

Search-engine queries

Because of the implications for privacy, search-engine queries are probably among the most difficult data to obtain. However, even if you do not work for a company that runs a search engine of its own, you may still find search-engine data in one of the following ways:

- Services such as Google Trends (trends.google.com) and Bing Search API (http://datamarket.azure.com/dataset/bing/search) provide indications of the number of times particular search terms were entered during certain time periods from various geographic areas. However, these are aggregated data, and only for terms that were queried with sufficient volume.

- Several companies install browser add-ons, known as *toolbars*, that allow them to collect data on users' browsing behaviors. They then sell these data after anonymization. One of the best-known of these companies is ComScore. The data collected by means of toolbars are very similar to the data to which a search engine's operator has access, albeit for a smaller population.

- We have had good experience generating our own search log by setting up a website with a mock search engine and having Mechanical Turk workers complete specific tasks.

Yahoo Answers

Yahoo Answers data can be obtained by means of the Yahoo application programming interface (developer.yahoo.com). The API allows users to query it for specific terms and to receive full question and answer text (and accompanying fields) in a structured output.

Yahoo's WebScope (webscope.sandbox.yahoo.com) is a highly developed academic collaboration program that makes datasets available for academic work.

Twitter

Twitter has had a love-hate relationship with the research community, at times prohibiting collation of Twitter datasets and at others allowing it or even encouraging these collections. At the time of writing, the easiest way to obtain a Twitter dataset is to purchase it from one of the companies authorized by Twitter to sell it.

Many people have created small datasets using the Twitter API (dev.twitter.com), but these may be more suitable for relatively focused information extraction tasks than for prospective analysis.

Web crawls

A Web crawl is essentially a copy of the visible Web. At the time of writing, the Web crawl offered by Common Crawl (commoncrawl.org) is the largest of its kind. The crawl is available through Amazon Web Services at http://aws.amazon.com/datasets/41740.

Dataset collections

As more and more data are collected, more datasets are made available. A few of my favorite locations for finding datasets are the following:

- Amazon Web Services (http://aws.amazon.com/datasets/)
- data provided by cities—for example, New York City (https://nycopendata.socrata.com/), Chicago (at https://data.cityof chicago.org/), Boston (at https://data.cityofboston.gov/), and Seattle (at https://data.seattle.gov/)

- databases of facts: http://www.freebase.com/, http://www.cyc
  .com/platform/opencyc, and http://wiki.dbpedia.org/Datasets
- other datasets: http://www.datawrangling.com/some-datasets-
  available-on-the-web/,   http://www.infochimps.com/,   and
  https://news.ycombinator.com/item?id=2165497

Notes

Introduction

1. The opening paragraph in *A Tale of Two Cities* reads: "It was the best of times, it was the worst of times, it was the age of wisdom, it was the age of foolishness, it was the epoch of belief, it was the epoch of incredulity, it was the season of Light, it was the season of Darkness, it was the spring of hope, it was the winter of despair, we had everything before us, we had nothing before us, we were all going direct to Heaven, we were all going direct the other way—in short, the period was so far like the present period, that some of its noisiest authorities insisted on its being received, for good or for evil, in the superlative degree of comparison only."

2. The National Security Agency collected data from nine major Internet companies, including Microsoft, Yahoo, Google, Facebook, PalTalk, AOL, Skype, YouTube, and Apple. See B. Gellman and L. Poitras, "U.S., British intelligence mining data from nine U.S. Internet companies in broad secret program," *Washington Post*, June 6, 2013 (available at http://wapo.st/1KzoPLK)

3. Google was fined for illegally collecting data from unencrypted Wi-Fi networks for its Google Street View project. See D. Graziano, "Google fined for illegal data collection," at http://bgr.com/2013/04/22/google -data-collection-germany-fine-456362/.

Chapter 1

1. "The Baruch Plan," presented to the United Nations Atomic Energy Commission June 14, 1946. See http://www.atomicarchive.com/Docs/ Deterrence/BaruchPlan.shtml.

2. The remaining 15 percent are mostly uninterested in the Internet or think it is too complicated. See http://pewinternet.org/Reports/2013/ Non-internet-users.aspx

3. Broadband connections have changed the way people use the Internet, moving them into more data-hungry activities such as video. The Pew Research Center, a USA Think Tank, documents how Americans use the Internet and how their use of it has changed. Pew reports are based on surveys of the U.S. population and so suffer from the drawbacks of self-reporting. Nevertheless, they are an extremely useful source for population-wide information on Internet use in the U.S. A recent survey of Internet use can be found at http://pewinternet.org/Static -Pages/Trend-Data-%28Adults%29/Online-Activites-Total.aspx.

4. ComScore pays people to install a toolbar, a small application that tracks how they use the Internet. ComScore publishes statistics on how people use the Internet from data collected in this way. For example, the statistics in this chapter are based on http://www.comscore.com/ Insights/Press_Releases/2013/1/comScore_Releases_December_2012 _U.S._Search_Engine_Rankings. What search engine someone uses is determined largely by what comes installed as the default search engine on a new computer, not by the quality of its results or by how easy it is to use. This "power of the default" is so strong that when the maker of the popular Firefox browser changed its default search engine from Google to Yahoo (in December of 2014), Yahoo's share of search queries increased by 2 percent in a single month. See http://www.businessinsider .com/google-firefox-message-yahoo-search-share-decline-2015-3.

5. Information on the amount of data that Facebook collects was provided in a technical note on the release of Corona (a software product, written by Facebook engineers, for scheduling the analysis of these

data). According to the technical note, Facebook collects approximately half a petabyte of information every day, or about 15 petabytes of data per month. Their data warehouse, where all these data are stored, grew by a factor of 2,500 between 2008 and 2012. The original technical note can be viewed at https://www.facebook.com/notes/facebook -engineering/under-the-hood-scheduling-mapreduce-jobs-more -efficiently-with-corona/10151142560538920. An analysis more accessible to laypersons can be found at http://www.theregister.co.uk/2012/ 11/09/facebook_open_sources_corona/.

6. I did not find official counts of the number of computers used by Amazon. The estimates I provide are of the number of publicly available computers on Amazon's public cloud, EC2. The estimate of half a million was derived by Huan Liu after some clever prodding of EC2—see http://www.enterprisetech.com/2014/11/14/rare-peek-massive-scale -aws/. Back-of-envelope estimates from information given at a talk by an Amazon executive provide the higher numbers—see http://www .enterprisetech.com/2014/11/14/rare-peek-massive-scale-aws/. One can only guess how many computers Amazon uses for its own needs and keeps hidden from the public.

7. Three words per query, a number often quoted in the search-engine industry, is based on a 2008 report by Yahoo. See, for example, Y. Song, H. Ma, H. Wang and K. Wang, "Exploring and exploiting user search behavior on mobile and tablet devices to improve search relevance," at http://research.microsoft.com/pubs/183843/fp016-songPS.pdf. Three words per query refers to queries submitted from desktop computers. Queries submitted from cell phones and other mobile devices tend to be shorter; in 2009 Google reported an average length of 2.44 words per query. Today, many people forgo text entry and use voice entry. In 2010, about 25 percent of users entered their queries via voice. See M. Shokouhi, R. Jones, U. Ozertem, K. Raghunathan, and F. Diaz, "Mobile query reformulations," in Proceedings of the 37th international ACM SIGIR Conference on Research & Development in Information Retrieval (ACM, 2014) (available at http://dl.acm.org/citation.cfm?id =2609497).

8. See C. Duhigg, "How companies learn your secrets," *New York Times*, February 16, 2012 (http://www.nytimes.com/2012/02/19/magazine/shopping-habits.html). The model used to predict which women were pregnant was the result of the work of Andrew Pole, a statistician working for Target.

9. According to data available at https://blog.compete.com/2009/10/22/bing-train-keeps-rolling-but-not-at-googles-expense/, Bing users make about 5 queries per day, significantly fewer than Google users (5.6) or Yahoo users (7.8). One of the reasons for this difference is, according to the source cited above, Bing's "promise to get users to answers quickly, in other words, with fewer searches."

10. L. Backstrom, J. Kleinberg, R. Kumar, and J. Novak, "Spatial Variation in Search Engine Queries" (http://www2008.wwwconference.org/papers/pdf/p357-backstromA.pdf). Events could also be localized in time as well as in space, and news events could be tracked. If you have ever wondered where the fan bases of various baseball teams are, see figure 8 in the paper.

11. Sakaki et al. were able to detect 96 percent of all earthquakes with an intensity of 3 or more on the Richter scale within a minute of their occurrence. See T. Sakaki, M. Okazaki, and Y. Matsuo, "Earthquake shakes Twitter users: Real-time event detection by social sensors," in *Proceedings of the 19th International Conference on World Wide Web* (ACM, 2010).

12. The term "infodemiology" was coined by G. Eysenbach in "Infodemiology and infoveillance: Framework for an emerging set of public health informatics methods to analyze search, communication and publication behavior on the Internet," *Journal of Medical Internet Research* 11 (2009), no. 1: e11.

13. G. Eysenbach, "Infodemiology: Tracking flu-related searches on the Web for syndromic surveillance," in AMIA Annual Symposium Proceedings 2006 (available at http://www.ncbi.nlm.nih.gov/pmc/articles/PMC1839505/). Eysenbach's advertisement was posted in response to queries containing "flu" or "flu symptoms" and read "Do you have the

flu? Fever, Chest discomfort, Weakness, Aches, Headache, Cough." The
ad contained a link to a generic patient-education website.

14. See J. Ginsberg et al., "Detecting influenza epidemics using search
engine query data," *Nature* 457, 2009: 1012–1014 (http://www.nature
.com/nature/journal/v457/n7232/abs/nature07634.html).The   Google
paper was, however, preceded by a lesser known paper: P. M. Polgreen,
Y. Chen, D. M. Pennock, and F. D. Nelson, "Using internet searches for
influenza surveillance," *Clinical Infectious Diseases* 47 (2008), no. 11:
1443–1448 (http://www.ncbi.nlm.nih.gov/pubmed/18954267). As an
example of the extent to which the latter is lesser known, consider that
as of this writing the Google paper has 1,517 citations and the paper by
Polgreen et al. has 241. Interestingly, today one could probably conduct
the same kind of research using the Google Trends website (http://
trends.google.com) without actual access to the query data. This is
because one does not need the individual searches, but only the number
of people who ask certain phrases. Those data are available on Google
Trends. If enough people ask for a specific term, Google Trends even
provides a geographic breakdown of searches.

15. People—and academic researchers are no exception—love to point
out other people's mistakes. There are a multitude of papers showing
Google's errors in predicting influenza prevalence. See, for example,
D. Butler, "When Google got flu wrong," *Nature* 494 (2013),
no. 7436: 155–156 (http://www.nature.com/news/when-google-got-flu
-wrong-1.12413).

16. See M. Barbaro and T. Zeller, "A face is exposed for AOL searcher
no. 4417749," *New York Times*, August 9, 2006. The searches that led
Barbaro and Zeller to Ms. Arnold were for "landscapers in Lilburn, Ga,"
several people with the last name Arnold, and "homes sold in shadow
lake subdivision Gwinnett county Georgia." These were not the only
searches Ms. Arnold made. For further details, see http://select.nytimes
.com/gst/abstract.html?res=F10612FC345B0C7A8CDDA10894DE4
04482.

17. See A. Narayanan, E. Shi, and B. Rubinstein, "Link prediction by
de-anonymization: How we won the Kaggle Social Network Challenge,"

in Proceedings of International Joint Conference on Neural Networks, 2011 (IEEE). "The goal of the contest," the authors write, "was to promote research on real world link prediction, and the dataset was a graph obtained by crawling the popular photo-sharing site Flickr, with users' identities scrubbed. By de-anonymizing much of the competition test set using our own Flickr crawl, we were able to effectively game the competition. Our attack represents a new application of de-anonymization to gaming machine learning contests, suggesting changes in how future competitions should be run." Addressing the wider problems of privacy, the authors write that their primary goal was "to raise attention to the ever-present possibility of de-anonymization in such contests." The full paper and a blog entry describing it are available at http://33bits.org/2011/03/09/link -prediction-by-de-anonymization-how-we-won-the-kaggle-social-network-challenge/.

18. C. Jernigan and B. Mistree, "Gaydar: Facebook friendships expose sexual orientation," *First Monday* 14 (2009), no. 10 (available at http://firstmonday.org/ojs/index.php/fm/article/viewArticle/2611/2302). "There is an old saying," Jernigan and Mistree write, "that "birds of a feather flock together." They continue: "The lesson is that people are self-segregating, such that the composition of your friends reflects on you. If the majority of your friends were male, one might predict you to be male. If many of your friends were a particular race, one might predict you to be that race. If many of your friends were gay, one might predict you to be gay. This predictive power works even though one knows nothing about you, as long as one knows something about your friends." Interestingly, in their paper Jernigan and Mistree show that more than 2 percent of friends of a sample of gay people were gay, versus fewer than 1 percent for the average heterosexual male.

19. The Office for Human Research Protections at the U.S. Department of Health and Human Services maintains a list of 96 countries with IRB-like bodies. The list is available at http://archive.hhs.gov/ohrp/international/HSPCompilation.pdf.

20. For a good overview of these principles, see R. Gillon, "Medical ethics: Four principles plus attention to scope," BMJ 309 (1994):184 (available at http://www.bmj.com/content/309/6948/184).

21. Katy Waldman reported on the experiment for *Slate*, writing that "Facebook intentionally made thousands upon thousands of people sad. Facebook's methodology raises serious ethical questions." See http://www.slate.com/articles/health_and_science/science/2014/06/ facebook_unethical_experiment_it_made_news_feeds_happier_or _sadder_to_manipulate.html.

22. Past research showed that such effects exist, but that research was based on much fewer samples and less comprehensive information on the structure of the social network. See J. H. Fowler and N. A. Christakis, "Dynamic spread of happiness in a large social network: Longitudinal analysis over 20 years in the Framingham Heart Study," BMJ 337 (2008): a2338 (available at http://www.bmj.com/content/337/bmj.a2338). The study by Fowler and Christakis is also controversial, albeit for other reasons. Interested readers are referred R. Lyons, "The spread of evidence-poor medicine via flawed social-network analysis," *Statistics, Politics, and Policy* 2 (2011) available at http://vw.slis.indiana.edu/talks-spring11/ Lyons.pdf).

23. Indeed, in an online survey conducted by the *Guardian* newspaper, 61 percent of respondents said they were not surprised by the Facebook experiment (http://www.theguardian.com/technology/poll/2014/jun/ 30/facebook-secret-mood-experiment-social-network). The value of such surveys is, however, questionable, since in the same survey 23 percent thought their feed was manipulated (though only 0.04 percent of users had their feed changed) and 66 percent said they considered closing their account. No noticeable decrease in Facebook use was apparent after the experiment.

24. People can rarely predict how users will behave in the presence of a new feature or service. For a few more examples of experiments and why they are needed, see R. Kohavi et al., "Trustworthy online controlled experiments: Five puzzling outcomes explained," in Proceedings of the 18th ACM SIGKDD International Conference on Knowledge Discovery and Data Mining, 2012 (available at http://robotics.stanford.edu/ users/ronnyk/puzzlingOutcomesInControlledExperiments.pdf).

25. As is well known, Google tested 41 shades of blue for the color of the toolbar on Google pages. See Laura M. Holson, "Putting a bolder

face on Google," *New York Times*, March 1, 2009 (available at http://
www.nytimes.com/2009/03/01/business/01marissa.html).

26. See, for example, G. A. Poland, R. M. Jacobson, and I. G. Ovsyan-
nikova, "Trends affecting the future of vaccine development and deliv-
ery: The role of demographics, regulatory science, the anti-vaccine
movement, and vaccinomics" *Vaccine* 27 (2009), no. 25–26: 3240–3244.

27. Michelle N. Meyer, "Everything you need to know about Facebook's
controversial emotion experiment," *Wired*, August 30, 2014 (available
at http://www.wired.com/2014/06/everything-you-need-to-know-about
-facebooks-manipulative-experiment/).

28. *The Economist* has also called for the use of electronic data to
improve health. See "Waiting on hold" (http://www.economist.com/
news/science-and-technology/21627557-mobile-phone-records-would-
help-combat-ebola-epidemic-getting-look). Referring to mobile telephone records, *The Economist* wrote: "Releasing the data, though, is not
just a matter for firms, since people's privacy is involved. It requires
government action as well. Regulators in each affected country would
have to order operators to make their records accessible to selected
researchers, who would have to sign legal agreements specifying how
the data may be used."

29. The OK Cupid blog contains quite a few interesting anecdotes for
cocktail-party talk, as well as for sociologists interested in human dating
behavior. The relevant blog entry is http://blog.okcupid.com/index.php/
the-biggest-lies-in-online-dating/. Christian Rudder, the author of the
blog and OK Cupid's chief scientist, recently published a book on his
observations. The book, titled *Dataclysm: Who We Are (When We Think
No One's Looking)*, gives spectacular insights into the dating behavior
of dating in the digital age. Another book in a similar vein is Oji Ogas
and Sai Gaddam, *A Billion Wicked Thoughts: What the Internet Tells Us
About Sexual Relationships*, which provides insights into sex-related
searches. As for people exaggerating their height to find spouses, there
are interesting examples of the opposite: In 1844, Adolphe Quetelet discovered that about 2 percent of French men reported being shorter than
was statistically expected, probably seeking to avoid conscription. See

Stephen M. Stigler, *The History of Statistics* (Harvard University Press, 1986), p. 215.

30. See P. Wicks, T. E. Vaughan, M. P. Massagli, and J. Heywood, "Accelerated clinical discovery using self-reported patient data collected online and a patient-matching algorithm," *Nature Biotechnology* 29 (2011): 411–414 (http://www.nature.com/nbt/journal/v29/n5/full/nbt .1837.html). "Although observational studies using unblinded data are not a substitute for double-blind randomized control trials," Wicks et al. write, "this study reached the same conclusion as subsequent randomized trials [on the use of Lithium for treatment of ALS], suggesting that data reported by patients over the internet may be useful for accelerating clinical discovery and evaluating the effectiveness of drugs already in use."

Chapter 2

1. F. J. Ingelfinger, "Arrogance," *New England Journal of Medicine* 303 (1980), no. 26: 1507–1511.

2. The paper describing this work is D. Pelleg, E. Yom-Tov, and Y. Maarek, "Can you believe an anonymous contributor? On truthfulness in Yahoo! Answers," in *Proceedings of the 2012 ASE/IEEE International Conference on Social Computing and 2012 ASE/IEEE International Conference on Privacy, Security, Risk and Trust* (IEEE, 2012).

3. See J. Cook, K. Kenthapadi, and N. Mishra, "Group chats on Twitter" (http://research.microsoft.com/pubs/184112/groupChatsOnTwitter-www2013.pdf). These group chats occur when a group of Twitter users agree on a time to meet and a hashtag (a key phrase) to identify messages related to the topic and discuss a topic of interest. There are group chats for a variety of topics. For health, the authors identified chats about addiction, mood disorders, and post-partum depression.

4. Another paper examining these questions is M. Kuebler et al., "When overweight is the normal weight: An examination of obesity using a social media internet database," *PLoS One* 8 (2013), no. 9: e73479.

5. R. S. Imes et al. show in "Patients' reasons for refraining from discussing internet health information with their healthcare providers" (http://www.tandfonline.com/doi/abs/10.1080/10410230802460580#.UrcApbTxW9k) that two reasons why patients do not discuss information they found on the Internet with their health-care providers are "fear of treading on the provider's turf" and "face-saving concerns."

6. See C. DeNavas-Walt, B. D. Proctor, and J. C. Smith, Income, Poverty, and Health Insurance Coverage in the United States: 2010, report issued by U.S. Department of Commerce (http://www.census.gov/prod/2011pubs/p60-239.pdf).

7. The problem of underinsurance is acute in the U.S. According to a Commonwealth Fund report titled "21 percent of adults with health insurance spent 5 percent or more of their income on out-of-pocket health care costs" (http://www.commonwealthfund.org/publications/press-releases/2014/nov/out-of-pocket-costs), 13 percent of adults with health insurance spend more than 10 percent of their income on health. That is comparable to that what most families spend on food (http://www.bls.gov/opub/btn/volume-2/spending-patterns-of-families-receiving-means-tested-government-assistance.htm). Underinsurance is a problem outside the U.S. too, and in many countries patients who suffer chronic illness or diseases that require expensive care are at much higher risk of poverty.

8. See R. R. White and E. Horvitz, "From Web search to healthcare utilization: Privacy-sensitive studies from mobile data," *Journal of the American Medical Informatics Association* 20 (2013), no. 1: 61–68(http://jamia.oxfordjournals.org/content/20/1/61). White and Horvitz tested the length of time between a query for symptom and a query that indicates utilization of health care, which they termed "evidence of health-care utilization." They even demonstrated that they could predict, from users' queries, whether users would seek medical attention.

9. These figures are based on results of a survey by the Pew Research Center summarized in "Health Online 2013" by S. Fox and M. Duggan and available at http://www.pewinternet.org/Reports/2013/Health-online/Summary-of-Findings.aspx. One of the interesting findings of

this survey pertains to the demographics of people who seek medical information online: These are more likely to be women, younger people, white adults, those who live in households earning $75,000 or more, and those with a college degree or advanced degrees.

10. R. R. White and E. Horvitz, "Cyberchondria: Studies of the escalation of medical concerns in web search" (http://research.microsoft.com/en-us/um/people/ryenw/papers/WhiteTOIS2009.pdf). The likelihood of having amyotrophic lateral sclerosis (ALS) is about 1 in 55,000 people. However, judging from information on the Web, about 7 percent of pages mention ALS as a reason for muscle twitching, though it is much more likely to be caused by one of a variety of very benign reasons. Similarly, the co-occurrence statistics for information from the Web may be interpreted naively by a searcher as indicating that there is a probability of 3 percent that "headache" is associated with "brain tumor," whereas in reality the incidence rate for a brain tumor is about 1 per 10,000 people.

11. J. K. Jerome, *Three Men in a Boat* (J. W. Arrowsmith, 1889).

12. The specific statistic is from W.D. Mosher, A. Chandra, and J. Jones, "Sexual behavior and selected health measures: Men and women 15–44 years of age, United States, 2002. Advance data from vital and health statistics," available at http://www.cdc.gov/nchs/data/ad/ad362.pdf. More (fascinating) data on sexual health can be found at http://www.iub.edu/~kinsey/resources/FAQ.html.

Chapter 3

1. According to http://www.myproana.com/index.php/topic/55581-one-meal-a-day/, myproana.com is "a site dedicated to the support or recovery of those suffering from eating disorders or body dysmorphic disorders." However, reading posts on this site make it clear that it is more about supporting eating disorders than about recovery.

2. We ran the queries "proana," "pro-anorexia," "thinspo," and "thinspiration" on October 27, 2013, using the Bing search engine. We

collected the returned results and listed sites that had "proana," "thin," "skinny," "anorexia," or "thinsp" in their addresses.

3. This is a quote from a blog called Proana Lifestyle (http:// proanalifestyle.blogspot.com); it has been removed. It is also the title of an article by S. Rainey in the *Telegraph* ("'Anorexia is a lifestyle, not a disease': An investigation into harrowing online forums promoting extreme dieting," February 25, 2014), an expose of online forums for anorexia. In the *Telegraph* article, Dr. Helen Sharpe, a professor at the Institute of Psychiatry at King's College London, is quoted as saying that these forums do not cause eating disorders but can perpetuate them. "What do they give people that they can't get elsewhere?" she asks. "Eating disorders can be extremely isolating conditions, and so finding a community of other people who think like you can be a powerful draw."

4. The quotation is from the front page of http://anabootcamp .weebly.com/. That website makes it clear that it is "for support for those with an eating disorder who feel alone and by themself with this issue." However, the site has sections that are likely to have a negative effect on anorexia sufferers, including one called "Thinspire" in which photos of emaciated women feature prominently.

5. Recommendation by the U.K. National Health Service, at http:// www.nhs.uk/chq/pages/1126.aspx?categoryid=51. The site recommends that "within a healthy, balanced diet, a man needs about 10,500 kJ (2,500 Kcal) a day to maintain his weight. For a woman, that figure is about 8,400 kJ (2,000 Kcal) a day."

6. According to http://www.jewishvirtuallibrary.org/jsource/Holocaust/ auconditions.htm: "Prisoners in the camp received meals three times a day: morning, noon, and evening. Factors influencing the nutritional value of the food included the official nutritional norms in the Nazi concentration camps. In practice, Auschwitz prisoners with less physically demanding labor assignments received approximately 1,300 calories per day, while those engaged in hard labor received approximately 1,700. After several weeks on such starvation rations in the camp, most prisoners began to experience organic deterioration that led to the

so-called "Muzulman" state, extreme physical exhaustion that ended in death."

7. This is quoted from a (since removed) blog called Proana Lifestyle (http://proanalifestyle.blogspot.com/2007/07/ways-to-hide-ed.html). This advice is listed on multiple proana sites on the Internet. Among the other tips on what to do before visiting a doctor are to drink water (to gain weight), to "dress warmly [so that your] temperature will be somewhat normal," and to "make sure [self-inflicted] wounds are healed." Tips for life at home and for visits with friends include "Go to bed early, you can't eat when you're asleep," "Take some cookies, or chips up to your room, and throw it away, then leave the empty packages in a place where parent will notice them," and "Tell people you are sooo hungry for a hamburger or something, then disappear, and when you return, tell them it was delicious!"

8. These tips are from http://www.myproana.com/index.php/topic/1689-pro-ana-tips-and-tricks/.

9. Source: http://diet.allwomenstalk.com/pro-ana-buddy-2/

10. The quotation is from an unattributed article in the *Daily Mail* titled "'Anorexia blogs nearly killed me': Even when Grainne, 17, was starving to death, 'thinspiration' sites encouraged her to lose more weight" (available at http://www.dailymail.co.uk/health/article-2398749/Pro-ana-Anorexia-blogs-nearly-killed-Starving-girl--17-says-thinspiration-sites-encouraged-her.html).

11. Adi Barkan is quoted in a BBC story titled "Israel passes law banning use of underweight models," available at: http://www.bbc.co.uk/news/world-middle-east-17450275. The Israeli law was proposed by Dr. Rachel Adato (then a member of the Knesset for the Kadima Party), Danny Dannon (a member of the Knesset for Likud), and Yael Latzer of Haifa University (an expert on eating disorders). Passing of laws similar to Israeli law was debated in the French Assembly and in the U.S. Congress, but has yet to be adopted outside Israel, owing in part to its implications for freedom of speech and freedom of occupation choice. And because the law was implemented only recently, it has not yet been shown to have caused a significant reduction in eating disorders.

12. The paper describing this work is E. Yom-Tov and d. boyd, "On the link between media coverage of anorexia and pro-anorexic practices on the Web," *International Journal of Eating Disorders* 47, no. 2 (2014): 196–202.

13. D. R. Cox's article "Regression models and life-tables" (*Journal of the Royal Statistical Society*, Series B, 34 (1972), no. 2: 187–220) is available at http://www.ida.liu.se/~kawah/Cox2.pdf.

14. Quoted in D. Goleman, "Pattern of death: Copycat suicides among youths," *New York Times*, March 18, 1987 (http://www.nytimes.com/ 1987/03/18/nyregion/pattern-of-death-copycat-suicides-among-youths .html). Although the article focuses on young people, they are by no means the only group of people amenable to the Werther Effect. D. P. Phillips documented adult suicides after suicide stories appeared in TV soap operas in "The impact of fictional television stories on U.S. adult fatalities: New evidence on the effect of the mass media on violence," *American Journal of Sociology* 87 (1982), no. 6: 1340–1359. However, several papers found no evidence for the Werther Effect in specific cases. See S. Platt, "The aftermath of Angie's overdose: is soap (opera) damaging to your health?" *British Medical Journal* 294 (1987): 954–957; G. Martin and L. Koo, "Celebrity suicide: Did the death of Kurt Cobain influence young suicides in Australia?" *Archives of Suicide Research* 3 (1997): 187–198.

15. The popular social networking site Tumblr tried to ban "thinspiration" content in March 2012. This was documented in an article by Nick Watts in the Huffington Post (available at http://www .huffingtonpost.co.uk/nick-watts/tumblr-thinspo-and-self-h_b _1382329.html). At the time we examined the number of queries that mentioned thinspiration and resulted in clicks to pages on Tumblr before and after the ban, and found no change in the number of queries. This is probably because even when content is banned, it quickly resurfaces under other names. As Watts wrote in his article, "While we can place these restrictions in our terms and conditions, remove blogs as and when they are found and remove users who are placing said content we can't stop the fact that it is there and it will always find its way online, even if it is only up for 24 hours. ... The only way we will ever

actually win against these issues is by not looking at the fire, but the fuel that keeps it going."

16. The paper describing this work is E. Yom-Tov, L. Fernandez-Luque, I. Weber, and S. P. Crain, "Pro-anorexia and pro-recovery photo sharing: A tale of two warring tribes," *Journal of Medical Internet Research* 14 (2012), no. 6: e151.

17. Source: http://www.flickr.com/photos/52322529@N02/5373480634/.

18. Source: comments on a photo of an apparently extremely underweight female a: http://www.flickr.com/photos/33465186@N04/41929 72020/. Interestingly, the other comment on this image, from another pro-anorexia user, is "Soo jealous!" Thus, users on Flickr receive both supportive comments and comments that view their condition as a disease to be treated.

19. C. Martijn et al., "Don't get the message: The effect of a warning text before visiting a proanorexia website," *International Journal of Eating Disorders* 42 (2009):139–145 (http://www.eetonderzoek.nl/publikaties/Martijn_2009_ijed.pdf). The warning label was aimed at first-time visitors to the site because, as the authors write, they did not expect regular visitors to proana sites "to change their behavior after reading our message. Rather, the warning text was written for new visitors who know nothing or very little about anorexia or proana." The label was a relatively lengthy explanation of proana and its consequences. Links to objective information about the disease were provided. About one third of users who saw the warning label decided not to continue to the pro-anorexia website—a huge effect for such a relatively minor intervention.

Chapter 4

1. See R. N. Proctor, "Commentary: Schairer and Schöniger's forgotten tobacco epidemiology and the Nazi quest for racial purity," *International Journal of Epidemiology* 30 (2001), no. 1: 31–34 (available at http://ije.oxfordjournals.org/content/30/1/31.extract).

2. On the history of Thalidomide, see http://www.sciencemuseum.org
.uk/broughttolife/themes/controversies/thalidomide.aspx.

3. See B. Fintel, A. T. Samaras, and E. Caria, "The Thalidomide tragedy:
Lessons for drug safety and regulation," *Helix*, July 28, 2009 (available at
http://scienceinsociety.northwestern.edu/content/articles/2009/
research-digest/thalidomide/title-tba).

4. Recently there have been claims that several of the popular diabe-
tes drugs approved by the FDA do not improve outcomes and have
caused several thousand deaths in the U.S. This has led to questions
about whether the approval process is rigorous and is measuring the
right outcomes. For a summary of the controversy, see Trudy Lieber-
man, "A closer look at the safety of FDA approved drugs," *Columbia
Journalism Review*, January 7, 2015 (available at http://www.cjr.org/the
_second_opinion/journal_sentinel_looks_closer_at_fda_approved_drugs
.php).

5. See, for example, http://en.wikipedia.org/wiki/Phases_of_clinical_
research and http://www.nlm.nih.gov/services/ctphases.html.

6. Source: S. U. Yasuda, L. Zhang, and S.-M. Huang, "The role of ethnicity in variability in response todrugs: Focus on clinical pharmacology
studies," *Clinical Pharmacology and Therapeutics* 84 (2008), no. 3:
417–423 (available at http://www.fda.gov/downloads/Drugs/Science
Research/ResearchAreas/Pharmacogenetics/UCM085502.pdf). This paper
lists multiple drugs the responses to which vary by ethnicity.

7. The URL of the FDA Adverse Event Reporting System (FAERS) is
http://www.fda.gov/Drugs/GuidanceComplianceRegulatoryInformation/
Surveillance/AdverseDrugEffects/default.htm. Adverse effects may be
reported to the FAERS MedWatch page: https://www.accessdata.fda.gov/
scripts/medwatch/. The FAERS website offers both the raw reports and
basic statistics on them.

8. For a summary of this work, see E. Yom-Tov and E. Gabrilovich,
"Postmarket drug surveillance without trial costs: Discovery of adverse
drug reactions through large-scale analysis of Web search queries," *Journal of Medical Internet research* 15, no. 6 (2013): e124.

9. It is always difficult to estimate what would have happened, but a large group of researchers led by W. G. van Panhuis tried to do just that ("Contagious diseases in the United States from 1888 to the present," *New England Journal of Medicine* 369, 2013, no. 22: 2151–2158). They tracked 56 diseases before and after vaccines were offered for them, and interpolated the number of cases that would be expected for those diseases had vaccines not been introduced. They found the mentioned reduction in the number of cases. For a summary of the paper, see Steve Lohr, "The vaccination effect: 100 million cases of contagious disease prevented," *New York Times*, November 27, 2013 (http://bits.blogs.nytimes.com/2013/11/27/the-vaccination-effect-100-million-cases-of-contagious-disease-prevented/?_r=2). The data for the article are available at http://www.tycho.pitt.edu/.

10. S. R. Owens, "Injection of confidence," *EMBO Reports* 3, no. 5 (2002): 406–409 (available at: http://www.ncbi.nlm.nih.gov/pmc/articles/PMC1084119/). Measles has spiked in the U.S. as well. An outbreak that started with a single case in December 2014 has, to date, caused 147 cases in seven states. The original case (the "index case") is unknown, but the virus is identical to the one that caused a measles outbreak in the Philippines in 2014. For more information, see http://www.cdc.gov/measles/multi-state-outbreak.html and http://www.cdc.gov/mmwr/preview/mmwrhtml/mm6406a5.htm?s_cid=mm6406a5_w.

11. John Snow's book, published in 1849, is titled *On the Mode of Communication of Cholera*. The second edition is available at http://books.google.com/books?id=-N0_AAAAcAAJ. The chapter dealing with the Broad Street pump is titled "The cholera near Golden Square." Snow's account of the incident is very readable and is quite frank about the limitations of his data.

12. A. M. Turing, "Computing machinery and intelligence," *Mind* 59, no. 236 (1950): 433–460.

13. H. A. Simon, *The Shape of Automation for Men and Management* (Harper & Row, 1965).

14. Source: Messaging, Malware and Mobile Anti-Abuse Working Group Report 15, 2011 (http://www.maawg.org/sites/maawg/files/news/

MAAWG_2011_Q1Q2Q3_Metrics_Report_15.pdf). Cisco estimated that in March 2014 more than 200 billion spam email messages were sent (http://blogs.cisco.com/security/spam-hits-three-year-high-water-mark)— about 77,000 per second! Spam filters are highly effective but not perfect, so even if one in a thousand spam messages is misclassified as legitimate 77 messages will pass the filter per second and will end up in someone's "in" mailbox.

15. See E. Yom-Tov et al., "Automatic identification of Web-based risk markers for health events," *Journal of Medical Internet Research* 17, no. 1 (2015): e29.

16. W.-K. Wong, A. Moore, G. Cooper, and M. Wagner, "WSARE: What's strange about recent events?" *Journal of Urban Health* 80 (2003), no. 1: i66–i75.

17. E. Yom-Tov, D. Borsa, I. J. Cox, and R. A. McKendry, "Detecting disease outbreaks in mass gatherings using Internet data," *Journal of Medical Internet Research* 16 (2014), no. 6: e154.

18. Kumbh Mela is considered the largest peaceful gathering on earth. The next largest gathering is the Shiite gathering at the shrine of Husayn ibn Ali in Iraq, which drew 20 million people in 2013.

Chapter 5

1. J. D. Bauby, *The Diving Bell and the Butterfly* (Knopf Group E-Books, 2008).

2. E. Kübler-Ross, *Coping with Death and Dying* (Ziff-Davis, 1973).

3. M. L. Stehl et al., "Conducting a randomized clinical trial of an psychological intervention for parents/caregivers of children with cancer shortly after diagnosis," *Journal of Pediatric Psychology* 34 (2009), no. 8: 803–816.

4. Y. Ofran et al., "Patterns of information-seeking for cancer on the Internet: an analysis of real world data." *PLoS One* 7, no. 9 (2012): e45921.

5. Several researchers have argued that the low pay of Mechanical Turk workers, which is sometimes well below the minimum wage in the U.S., amounts to exploitation. See, e.g., G. Norcie, "Ethical and practical considerations for compensation of crowdsourced research participants," CHI Workshop on ethics logs and videotape: Ethics in large scale trials & user generated content, 2011 (available at http://www.crowdsourcing.org/document/ethical-and-practical-considerations-for-compensation-of-crowdsourced-research-participants/3650).

6. See, e.g., the Mayo Clinic's Web page on thyroid cancer (http://www.mayoclinic.org/diseases-conditions/thyroid-cancer/basics/definition/CON-20043551). This page has the following sections: Symptoms, Causes, Risk factors, Complications, Preparing for your appointment, Tests and diagnosis, Treatment and drugs, Coping and support, and Prevention. For a patient already diagnosed, the first three sections are superfluous; so, probably, are the next two. Only two of the sections are of interest to such people. (The Mayo Clinic is not unique in this respect; many of the pages on diseases, especially more serious ones, have the same format as the one outlined here.) Knowing the status of a person with regard to the disease can help serve more relevant content to individuals.

7. The quotation is from a talk by Gary Greenberg presented on the Australian Broadcasting Corporation's *Big Ideas* program in December 2013. Audio of the talk is available at http://www.abc.net.au/radionational/programs/bigideas/psychiatry-under-the-microscope/5134818. Greenberg's views are summarized in *The Book of Woe: The DSM and the Unmaking of Psychiatry* (Blue Rider, 2013).

8. The quotation is from Lovelace's 2008 book *Scattershot: My Bipolar Family* (Dutton).

9. See E. Yom-Tov, R.W. White, and E. Horvitz, "Seeking insights about cycling mood disorders via anonymized search logs," *Journal of Medical Internet Research* 16 (2014), no. 2: e65.

10. M. De Choudhury, S. Counts, E. J. Horvitz, and A. Hoff, "Characterizing and predicting postpartum depression from shared Facebook

data," in *Proceedings of the 17th ACM conference on Computer supported cooperative work & social computing* (ACM, 2014). It is important to note that although Facebook posts are predictive of postpartum depression, their accuracy is far from that needed for a medical system to operate independently. In an article in the *New York Times* (Natasha Singer, "Risks in using social media to spot signs of mental distress," December 26, 2014), Mark Eredze of Johns Hopkins University was quoted as saying: "People always ask 'Can you predict who is going to commit suicide? I think that's way beyond what anyone can do."

11. See Michelle Starr, "Samaritans Radar depression app raises Twitter privacy concerns," CNET, November 3, 2014 (http://www.cnet.com/news/samaritans-radar-depression-app-raises-twitter-privacy-concerns/). Starr expressed concern that Twitter was making too many assumptions: "that everyone on Twitter is friends with all their followers, or that they'd be OK with every single one of their followers being alerted that they're suicidal every time that they mention they're depressed—even in jest," "that everyone using the app has the best intentions," and that "it only monitors public Tweets."

12. See, for example, M. A. Hamburg and F. S. Collins, "The path to personalized medicine," *New England Journal of Medicine* 363 (2010), no. 4: 301–304.

Epilogue

1. For example, researchers have linked searches for fruits and vegetables and (separately) searches for alcohol consumption to risk for chronic disease at a state-wide level in the U.S. See T. Nguyen et al., "Web search activity data accurately predict population chronic disease risk in the USA," *Journal of Epidemiology and Community Health* 69 (2015), no. 7: 693–699.

2. Published in the September 1956 issue of *Astounding Science Fiction*.

Index